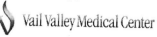

STRESS
MANAGEMENT
INTERVENTION
—— for Women With ——
Breast Cancer

STRESS
MANAGEMENT
INTERVENTION
—— for Women With ——
Breast Cancer

MICHAEL H. ANTONI

With Contributions by
Roselyn Smith

American Psychological Association • Washington, DC

Published by
American Psychological Association
750 First Street, NE
Washington, DC 20002
www.apa.org

To order
APA Order Department
P.O. Box 92984
Washington, DC 20090-2984

Tel: (800) 374-2721, Direct: (202) 336-5510
Fax: (202) 336-5502, TDD/TTY: (202) 336-6123
On-line: www.apa.org/books/
E-mail: order@apa.org

In the U.K., Europe, Africa, and the Middle East, copies may be ordered from
American Psychological Association
3 Henrietta Street
Covent Garden, London
WC2E 8LU England

Typeset in Meridien by AlphaWebTech, Mechanicsville, MD

Printer: United Book Press, Baltimore, MD
Cover Designer: Naylor Design, Washington, DC
Technical/Production Editors: Jennifer Powers and Jennifer L. Macomber

The opinions and statements published are the responsibility of the authors, and such opinions and statements do not necessarily represent the policies of the American Psychological Association.

Library of Congress Cataloging-in-Publication Data

Antoni, Michael H.
   Stress management intervention for women with breast cancer / By
Michael H. Antoni and Roselyn G. Smith.
       p. cm.
Includes bibliographical references and index.
    ISBN 1-55798-941-9
    1. Breast—Cancer—Psychological aspects. 2. Stress management for
women. I. Smith, Roselyn. II. Title.

RC280.B8 A585 2002
616.99'449'0019—dc21   2002015843

British Library Cataloguing-in-Publication Data
A CIP record is available from the British Library.

Printed in the United States of America
First Edition

This book is dedicated to the hundreds of thousands of women who are dealing with breast cancer in this country and to the leagues of others who are challenged with this disease each year around the world. It is our hope that the techniques that we have assembled, tailored, taught, and tested with these women in the weeks after their surgery have lasting effects on their ability to manage the ongoing stress of their diagnosis and treatment. We further hope that these techniques may help them to somehow use this period in their lives to mobilize their inner strengths, enhance their sense of purpose, and enrich the personal relationships that have been so important in supporting them through all of these challenges and shall be important for future ones to come.

Contents

5

Preface

For more than a decade, we have examined ways to help women deal with the experience of having breast cancer. Initially, we examined relationships among stress, coping, and personality variables in women who were receiving a diagnosis and undergoing surgery for early-stage breast cancer. Subsequently, we expanded our focus to investigate the effects of psychosocial intervention during the months after surgery in women with early-stage breast cancer and to explore predictors of quality of life in long-term survivors of cancer.

During the past several years, we have tested the efficacy of psychosocial intervention as a means of facilitating adjustment during the initial months after surgery, when women are beginning physically demanding adjuvant therapies such as chemotherapy and radiation treatments. Newer studies are also testing the effects of the intervention during the months after adjuvant therapy has ended, a time when many women are gripped with anxiety and fears about disease recurrence on one hand and the challenges of resuming their life responsibilities on the other. We are currently in the process of developing this intervention for Spanish-speaking women and those from other ethnic minority groups in the hopes of creating an intervention that is effective for as many women with breast cancer as possible. All research was conducted at the University of Miami: the Department of Psychology, the Center for Psycho-Oncology Research, and the Sylvester Cancer Center.

Our theoretical frame of reference holds that appropriate patient management of women with breast cancer can facilitate psychological adjustment to diagnosis and treatment challenges and might also reduce the likelihood of disease recurrence. Interventions targeting optimal disease management are usually classified as secondary prevention approaches and are designed to prevent any psychological or physical complications of extant disease. We reasoned that an efficient way to address secondary prevention issues was to think of breast cancer as a chronic disease that could be affected by biological, behavioral, and psychosocial phenomena. Through a series of prospective studies of women in the various diagnosis and treatment periods for breast cancer, we determined that psychological factors such as optimism, certain coping strategies, and social support could substantially affect the ways in which women adjusted to and actually thrived during diagnosis, surgery, and adjuvant therapy. Drawing from this work, we determined that one way to intervene was to develop a group-based cognitive–behavioral stress management (CBSM) program that could directly improve quality of life, improve immune functioning, and possibly prevent disease recurrence.

First, we thought that CBSM could improve quality of life by decreasing the distress and depressed affect associated with having a chronic and life-threatening disease, increasing the use of adaptive cognitive coping strategies (e.g., acceptance, positive reframing), and increasing or maintaining social support resources. Second, we believed that CBSM could also decrease women's use of avoidance and denial as coping strategies. We also reasoned that, similar to people with other chronic diseases (such as HIV infection), women who were encouraged to use problem-focused rather than emotion-focused coping in appropriate situations would have an enhanced sense of self-efficacy and self-esteem. Third, we thought that a CBSM intervention that included relaxation training might be able to attenuate the impact of stressors on stress hormone levels (e.g., cortisol) and the immune system and in so doing might decrease the likelihood of disease recurrence.

We conceptualized breast cancer as (a) a chronic disease with a clinical course that could be affected by multiple behavioral and biological factors and (b) a chronic stressor that creates multiple burdens at the psychological and physical levels—burdens that may overwhelm an individual's coping resources. We reasoned that women who have recently received a diagnosis of breast cancer are among the individuals who might benefit substantially from interventions that teach them to cope with such ongoing demands. We banked on the notion that using an intervention such as CBSM to help women develop good coping skills and a strong sense of coping self-efficacy would increase psychological adjustment and stress resistance, which could reduce the chances of disease recurrence.

This text describes how we developed, validated, and implemented one CBSM intervention, the *Breast Cancer Stress Management And Re-*

laxation *Training* (B-SMART) program for women dealing with breast cancer. It is our hope that this volume will allow clinicians to use this program with their patients and duplicate some of the very encouraging results that we have documented during our validation studies. We also hope that clinical researchers will be motivated to use this volume and will formulate new ways to apply the B-SMART approach to studies that explore ways to optimize the quality of life and physical health of people with cancer.

Acknowledgments

We are very grateful for and have been entirely dependent on the time, courage, commitment, and unrelenting effort that hundreds of women have offered to our research program during the past 10 years. They allowed us to peer into their daily lives while they managed one of their most substantial challenges ever—receiving a diagnosis of breast cancer, undergoing surgery, and receiving adjuvant therapy. They told us about their major fears, concerns, and frustrations and what it was like shortly after getting the news of the diagnosis; during the days before surgery; and during the weeks after surgery, when they mourned their losses and anxiously anticipated the physical and emotional challenges of chemotherapy and radiation. They told us about how they remained optimistic; about their behavioral and cognitive coping techniques; and how they sought out help from their spouses, partners, family members, and friends. We learned that some women drew their major support from spouses, whereas others used female family members or people from their religious and spiritual world. We responded by assembling the best available stress management techniques possible. We tailored them to address the women's primary concerns and delivered them in the form of a supportive group composed of female group leaders and women with breast cancer. We only hope that the B-SMART program begins to repay the debt that we owe these women for all of these efforts.

We are also indebted to the families, friends, and extended support networks of these women, people who let us intrude into their private lives long enough to learn about the ways these supportive networks can influence women's adjustment to this extremely challenging period. It would have been very easy for these people to try to "protect" the women from research studies to preserve their privacy. Instead, we were overwhelmed with the courage of and insights from spouses, family members, and friends. They encouraged women to enroll in our studies, patiently waited while they filled out lengthy questionnaires in their homes, and then helped drive them to group sessions and follow-up assessment visits. Their efforts have helped us complete all the steps necessary to validate the B-SMART program, and now it can be used confidently by scores of other women going through the experience of having breast cancer.

The tailoring and validation of the B-SMART program would not have been possible without the unselfish cooperation of the surgeons, oncologists, and nurses who referred their patients to us from clinics, hospitals, and cancer centers during the years of our studies. This often required them to take hours out of their busy schedules to promote our studies to their patients, allow us to place recruitment flyers in their waiting rooms, and help us keep track of the women as they progressed through various stages in their treatment and recovery. They did all of this without a dime of reimbursement. In this era in which the quantity of health care is often determined by the "bottom line," we are greatly impressed with their generosity. We are especially indebted to Robert Dehrogopian, a surgical oncologist who referred numerous women to us for the clinical trials evaluating the B-SMART program.

The research necessary to develop and test the B-SMART intervention would not have been possible without the rich and creative theoretical framework laid out by Charles S. Carver, a trailblazer in the psychology of breast cancer at the University of Miami and one of the founders of this line of research in the field of behavioral medicine during the late 1980s and early 1990s. His theoretical work on the role of optimism and coping in the context of stress and disease and his development of contemporary measurement instruments to monitor these constructs during this early period were critical in providing the scientific scaffolding necessary to assemble, tailor, and test what is now the B-SMART program. Dr. Carver also played a key role in managing the large teams of graduate students and postdoctoral fellows that we needed to collect, analyze, and publish all of the data. His current work, developing instruments designed to monitor the quality of life of patients who are classified as long-term survivors, will allow us to track the long-term benefits that women maintain up to a decade after they have completed the B-SMART program.

We are very thankful for the many weeks, months, semesters, and years that our teams of undergraduates, graduate students, postdoctoral fellows, and faculty and staff members have dedicated to this program of research. This team of researchers worked many long hours recruiting patients through doctors' offices and community events; conducting telephone screens; visiting patients at their homes, jobs, and clinics; and running group sessions until late at night and on weekends. They then worked at the computer for the rest of the night or weekend, entering data and crunching the statistics that would tell us how well this intervention worked. Many of the results of this work were drawn from numerous theses and dissertations that the members of this research team carefully crafted, presented at scientific meetings around the world, and ultimately published in scientific journals. We hope that these experiences were as rewarding for our students as they were for their proud professors. The individuals constituting our research team during the past decade have included faculty members such as Gail Ironson, Ron Duran, Bonnie Blomberg, Sharlene Weiss, and Charles Carver as well as our coinvestigator in the immunology laboratory, Maria Romero; postdoctoral fellows including Suzanne Harris, Susan Yount, Kristin Kilbourn, Yvonne Hinkle, Amy Boyers, Dean Cruess, Alicea Price, Stacy Spencer, Suzanne Lechner, and Tammy Enos; and graduate students including Susan Alferi, Kristi Pozo-Kaderman, Vida Petronis, Bonnie McGregor, Roselyn Smith, Sophie Gellati, Cassy Vaughn, Kenya Murphy, Therese West, Kurrie Wells, Jessica Lehman, Jenifer Culver, Pati Arena, and Christina Wynings. Finally, we are greatly indebted to three of our staff members, Janny Rodriquez, Linda Kahan, and Lynne Hudgins, who helped make our studies run smoothly, took great care of all the women participating in our research studies, and kept our funding agencies happy. We further acknowledge Lynne Hudgins for doing the lion's share of the clerical work necessary to bring this volume to fruition.

We would like to express our respectful gratitude to the state and federal funding agencies that have provided the continued support necessary to keep our research program in operation for the past several years. In the late 1980s and early 1990s, the American Cancer Society was a major force in supporting the research studies that provided the theoretical basis for the development of the B-SMART program. During the mid-1990s, the U.S. Department of Defense was a major source of funding for training of our graduate students to conduct this research during their 4-year posts at the university. Since 1992, the National Cancer Institute (NCI) has been the major source of support for the studies that tailored, revised, and validated the current form of the B-SMART program. The support has involved the funding of empirical research on more than 400 women during the period of diagnosis, surgery, and adjuvant therapy for breast cancer. The NCI is supporting our current research, which is designed to test the effects of this intervention in women who have recently completed their adjuvant therapy and women who have received the intervention in Spanish. The NCI is also supporting our studies of long-term survivors of cancer, which will, among other things, test how the B-SMART intervention influences the long-term psychological and physical health of women with breast cancer by tracking B-SMART participants up to a decade after they have completed the program. We and all of the women who are present and future beneficiaries of the B-SMART program owe a great deal to these funding institutions.

STRESS
MANAGEMENT
INTERVENTION
— for Women With —
Breast Cancer

Introduction

Each year almost 200,000 women are diagnosed with breast cancer in the United States alone. Moments after each of these hundreds of thousands of diagnoses are given by physicians, the women on the receiving end suddenly leave the healthy world and become patients–and run face-to-face into a major life crisis. "How bad is it, and what are my options? What are the side effects of the best treatments available? Will I ever be the same again, or will I be just a part of who I am now? How will my husband or partner think about me? Will I live to see my kids grow up? Will I be able to spend future holidays with my grandchildren?" These are only a few of the questions that these women ask themselves and their physicians after they learn they have breast cancer, even when it is caught in the earliest stages.

Individuals dealing with breast cancer experience continual psycho-social stressors including fears of recurrence and concerns about physical deterioration during adjuvant therapies such as radiation and chemo-therapy (Spencer et al., 1999). Inadequately coping with these demands may lead to depressed affect, hostility, reduced use of social supports, substance abuse, impaired immune functioning, and possibly accelerated disease progression.

Although initial research suggested that severe emotional reactions to cancer diagnosis and initial treatment are common among patients with breast cancer, more recent work suggests the importance of think-ing of cancer-related distress along a continuum of adjustment ranging from mild distress to severe symptoms of depressive and anxiety disorders. Today, most consider the diagnosis and treatment of breast cancer to be a crisis, but the experience is spread out over the period of a year for most women with early-stage cancer (i.e., women with a favorable prognosis). However, some women may experience the diagnosis and treatment as more traumatic and display symptoms of posttraumatic stress disorder or other anxiety- and depressive-related conditions. In many women, anxiety and depressive symptoms persist for 4 to 5 months, yet even at subclinical levels they can affect their quality of life after surgery for breast cancer. In addition to affecting quality of life, cancer-related distress may cause additional visits to physicians' offices and to hospitals, interfere with treatment decision making, and disrupt ongoing curative and adjuvant treatments—which can increase costs and increase the burden on caregivers, resulting in caregiver burnout.

All of these issues can eventually erode a woman's social support network. This book explains the techniques psychologists have developed to help women move through this period with minimal levels of disruption. In some cases, they can actually benefit from the situation— it can become a positive, life-changing experience. In particular, we focus on the theoretical rationale and empirical validation of a psychosocial intervention designed specifically for women dealing with the diagnosis and treatment for breast cancer: the *Breast Cancer Stress Management And Relaxation Training*, or B-SMART, program.

As a prelude to developing the B-SMART program, we spent years interviewing women in the weeks before and months after their breast cancer diagnosis, surgery, and adjuvant therapy. We explored their chief concerns, how they adjusted psychologically to these experiences, and which psychosocial factors helped them the most as them attempted to manage this stressful period. We found that their chief concerns involve fears of recurrence, concerns about being sick or damaged by adjuvant therapy, not seeing children grow up, premature death, life with their partner being cut short, and loss of sexual desirability and sexual feelings. These issues can predict emotional distress, sexual disruption, and impairments in sense of femininity. We have also found that the types and severity of concerns about breast cancer seem to vary as a function of ethnicity, personality factors—such as optimism and investment in body image and body integrity as sources of self-acceptance, and external resources such as social support. We also know that women differ substantially in the degree to which these concerns cause distress and disrupt their quality of life. The women who are most resilient seem to be those who use particular coping strategies, such as positive reframing or relying on religion, and those who have social support from family and friends.

Importantly, each of these coping strategies can vary according to contextual factors such as the woman's religious affiliation and marital status. For instance, we know that the use of religion as a coping strategy seems to most effectively buffer distress among woman who are Protestant. Women with high levels of social support from their spouses and female family members may experience less distress after surgery than more isolated women; however, certain types of support (e.g., material or instrumental support) from certain sources (e.g., female family members) may be detrimental. We have also learned that social support, especially support from female family members, tends to erode over time among women who remain distressed about their breast cancer for a long time after the diagnosis. Thus, numerous complex factors are involved in determining just the right mix of coping strategies and resources for helping a woman adjust to breast cancer.

In addition to clarifying these complexities, these findings highlighted the value of using psychosocial intervention, particularly group-based cognitive–behavioral intervention, to facilitate the adjustment process during the period after diagnosis and initial treatment for breast cancer. Cognitive coping responses and positive thinking are a prime example. If an intervention could teach women to use coping strategies such as positive reframing and to maintain a more optimistic outlook, they might experience less distress after diagnosis and surgery. These findings also highlighted the need to focus on maintenance and enhancement of social contacts. We reasoned that interventions teaching skills such as assertiveness could assist women in telling family and friends which of their actions were helpful and which were not. We also decided that a group-based intervention format was crucial because the group itself could serve as a source of emotional support. A supportive group should help women resist the urge to withdraw from other sources of support and aspects of normal life. Hence, this program focuses not only on providing support but also on teaching cognitive–behavioral techniques to help participants increase or maintain social support and change their outlook toward the future.

To date, our research program has documented the specific concerns that patients with breast cancer have in the weeks after surgery and how age and ethnicity influence these concerns. We have used this information to tailor the focus of the B-SMART program, a program that is described in great detail in this book. We have documented that women assigned to the B-SMART program have a lower prevalence of depression and an increase in a sense of positive growth coming from the cancer experience. We also showed that these psychological changes were accompanied by decreases in physiological arousal as indicated by decreases in serum cortisol levels. Finally, women in the B-SMART program showed improvements in immune cell functioning, which could decrease their risk of cancer recurrence. Our research program is now tracking these women for a 5-year period to determine whether women completing the B-SMART program enjoy continued improvements in quality of life, a longer disease-free interval, and increased survival time.

Stress Management Intervention for Women With Breast Cancer is targeted for clinicians and clinical researchers dealing with psychosocial issues of women diagnosed with breast cancer. On the basis of more than 10 years of funded research, the stress management program described in this book comprises a blend of empirically supported cognitive–behavioral stress management (CBSM) techniques that have been tailored to the special needs of women dealing with the stress of breast cancer and its treatment. This stress management program has been designed to be used by mental health professionals such as clinical psychologists, psychiatrists, social workers, and nurses.

This book is divided into a textbook portion and the *Therapist's Manual* used in the B-SMART program. There is also a *Participant's Workbook*. In chapter 1 of the textbook, I describe the rationale for the use of CBSM with individuals diagnosed with and treated for breast cancer. Chapter 2 includes the experimental evidence validating the efficacy of this CBSM intervention in different cohorts of patients with breast cancer; I also outline ongoing investigations. In chapter 3, I provide an overview of the B-SMART program, a time-limited CBSM intervention protocol we standardized on and adapted to the challenges facing these women. In chapter 4, I describe the steps and special considerations involved in clinically implementing the intervention and include several case examples. In chapter 5, I review the issues and procedures available for assessing progress and treatment outcomes in the intervention.

The *Therapist's Manual* is used to deliver the CBSM B-SMART intervention. The manual is organized into 10 weekly sessions comprising a 90-minute CBSM portion and a 45-minute relaxation and imagery portion. Each session contains an outline listing materials and preparations needed to conduct the session; a stated goal; various relevant examples, such as frequently encountered target stressors, stressor appraisals, coping responses, adaptive and maladaptive behaviors, and models and steps for behavior change; in-session exercises that use imagery, behavioral role-playing, and group sharing; and instructions for using take-home exercises and self-monitoring materials.

The *Participant's Workbook* is given to women who are participating in the B-SMART program. The workbook contains a summary of each of the 10 intervention session and includes suggested out-of-session homework assignments that can be used to solidify the material introduced in the weekly sessions. The workbook also includes complete sets of self-monitoring materials (e.g., stressor diary sheets, relaxation exercises, sleep monitoring sheets).

Stress Management for Women With Breast Cancer

1

How does one begin to choose and evaluate the most efficacious interventions for women dealing with breast cancer? Establishing the efficacy of psychosocial interventions to optimize quality of life and physical health outcomes in patients with cancer has been of great interest to clinical researchers in the field of psycho-oncology for more than 30 years.

Psycho-oncology can be considered a subdiscipline of health psychology. It encompasses basic and applied research examining how psychosocial and biobehavioral factors influence cancer risk and health maintenance behaviors, as well as research of the factors associated with the development of, adjustment to, and clinical course of human cancers. Because of the potentially wide-ranging influence of such psychosocial and biobehavioral factors, investigators and clinical practitioners involved in psycho-oncology often specialize in one area of this subdiscipline. Specialization may include work that involves identifying and intervening with factors associated with (a) the onset and maintenance of cancer risk behaviors such as cigarette smoking, poor diet, and ultraviolet light exposures or cancer prevention behaviors such as mammography exams or risk factor screening; (b) the initiation and subclinical promotion of cancer development; (c) the adjustment to a diagnosis of and medical treatment for cancer; and (d) the progression of, recurrence of, or survival from an extant cancer.

Each one of these areas of psycho-oncology includes diverse research that has applied numerous psychological theories—ranging from psychodynamic to social learning to classical conditioning theories—to address the risk for developing cancer, poorly adjusting to a cancer diagnosis, or a poor health course after treatment. Our research during the past 10 years, most of which has been funded by the National Cancer Institute and the American Cancer Society, has focused on better understanding the association among psychosocial phenomena, physiological regulatory mechanisms, biological processes, and health outcomes in patients with or at risk for the development of specific cancers. This book summarizes this decade of research as it applies to the study of breast cancer, work that has culminated in the development and evaluation of an intervention specifically designed to improve quality of life and physical health of women diagnosed with breast cancer—the *Breast Cancer Stress Management And Relaxation Training* (B-SMART) program.

Psychosocial Factors: Adjustment to Breast Cancer Diagnosis and Treatment

HOW DO WOMEN ADJUST TO A DIAGNOSIS OF BREAST CANCER?

Early research suggested that severe emotional reactions to cancer diagnosis and initial treatment are common among patients with breast cancer (Derogatis et al., 1983; Meyerowitz, 1980; P. Miller, 1980), although subsequent work indicated that severe symptoms are unlikely if no prior psychiatric disorder exists (Bloom, 1987; Gordon et al., 1980; Irvine, Brown, Crooks, Roberts, & Browne, 1991; Lansky et al., 1985; Penman et al., 1987; van't Spijker, Trijsberg, & Duivenvoorden, 1997). A contemporary view of reactions to cancer suggests the importance of conceptualizing cancer-related distress along a continuum of adjustment that ranges from mild distress to severe variants of depressive and anxiety disorders (Holland, 2000). One prospective study that researched women throughout their treatment for breast cancer revealed that anxiety and depressive symptoms persist for a 4- to 5-month period and decrease a woman's quality of life (Longman, Braden, & Mishel, 1999).

Beyond affecting quality of life, cancer-related distress may cause additional visits to physicians' offices and hospitals, interfere with treatment decisions, and disrupt ongoing curative and adjuvant treatments, resulting in increased costs of care and caregiver burden and burnout (Holland, 2000). Not all patients experience equal levels of distress at the same point during the disease process. This has prompted behavioral researchers to examine individual differences in cancer perceptions and in contextual and personality factors that are associated with adjustment in different people with cancer. During the past few years, psycho-oncology researchers have identified factors associated with psychosocial adjustment to numerous types of cancer. Among these types of cancer, we have learned the most about women diagnosed with breast cancer.

PRIMARY CONCERNS OF WOMEN WITH BREAST CANCER

Today the dominant view about the experience of having breast cancer is that being diagnosed and treated constitute crises in the lives of women who experience them, but the experience spans a year by most women with the early stage of the disease (i.e., women with a favorable prognosis). However, some women may feel the diagnosis and treatment are more traumatic and display some symptoms of posttraumatic stress disorder (PTSD; Cordova, Studts, Hann, Jacobsen, & Andrykowski, 2000). The chief concerns of women with breast cancer involve fears of recurrence; concerns about being sick or damaged by adjuvant therapy; not being with their children as they grow up; premature death; early menopause; life with their partner being cut short; and loss of attractiveness, sexual desirability, and sexual feelings (Spencer et al., 1999). These issues make unique contributions to predicting emotional distress, sexual disruption, and impairments in feelings of femininity in these women as well. In two separate groups of women (n = 144 and 202), patients with early-stage breast cancer who expected to remain cancer free in the future reported less emotional distress (Carver, Harris, et al., 2000). It also appears that there are significant ethnic differences in the concerns reported and the adverse reactions expressed by patients with breast cancer (Spencer et al., 1999). Hispanic women report more intense concerns than do other women, as well as higher levels of emotional distress and social and sexual disruptions, whereas African American women report lower levels of distress and disruption in sense of femininity than the other groups (Spencer et al., 1999). The results of this research are summarized in chapter 2. In addition to individual differences in adjustment that are attributable to ethnicity, we are also learning that specific personality and contextual factors may also predict how a woman will adjust during the breast cancer treatment experience.

PERSONALITY FACTORS

Personality factors involved in the ways the cancer experience is appraised may also affect adjustment and quality of life among women with breast cancer. One of these dimensions is optimism versus pessimism (Carver et al., 1993). This variable (which is assessed before surgery) predicts emotional distress at several points during the year after surgery in patients with breast cancer.

How does being optimistic protect women from being distressed? Evidence shows that the effects are a result of different coping strategies. Specifically, greater acceptance as a coping strategy predicts lower distress, whereas the use of disengagement predicts more distress after surgery. Disengagement also appears to mediate the effects of pessimism on the development of distress up to 6 months after surgery. These findings are similar to those from another study involving patients with breast cancer who were assessed before and after undergoing breast biopsies and 3 weeks after surgery (Stanton & Snider, 1993). Together these studies suggest that certain kinds of coping responses are important in their own right, a conclusion supported by other recent prospective studies of coping in patients with breast cancer (Heim, Valach, & Schaeffner, 1997). It also suggests that patients with cancer may benefit from the opportunity to modify cognitive appraisals (i.e., increase optimism and use of acceptance and positive reframing through cognitive restructuring and coping-skills training) in the context of a psychosocial intervention.

Other constructs closely related to optimism and pessimism, such as helplessness, hopelessness, and a giving-up attitude, have been widely studied in patients with cancer (e.g., Greer et al., 1992). The degree to which these individual variables reflect coping responses versus dispositional personality traits is still up for debate. Nevertheless, interventions that are able to change these characteristics among people dealing with cancer are likely to contribute to improvements in quality of life. Some work also suggests that patients with breast cancer with greater levels of helplessness and hopelessness may be at heightened risk for disease relapse (Watson, Haviland, Greer, Davidson, & Bliss, 1999). This suggests that psychosocial interventions may be able to affect disease relapse rates in patients with breast cancer by altering their perceptions about their own abilities (i.e., by replacing feelings of helplessness with feelings of increased self-efficacy) and their future (i.e., by replacing a sense of hopelessness with optimism).

CONTEXTUAL FACTORS

Many researchers have examined contextual factors related to variations in adjustment among patients with cancer. One such variable is adequacy of social support. Patients who think that they have inadequate support fare worse than those who think that they have adequate support (e.g., Bloom, 1982, 1986; Funch & Mettlin, 1982; Helgeson & Cohen, 1996; Irvine et al., 1991; Jamison, Wellisch, & Pasnau, 1978; Meyerowitz, 1980; Northouse, 1988; Vachon, 1986; Wortman, 1984). The crisis of cancer can overwhelm a spouse or significant other, eroding the person's ability to be supportive (Bolger, Foster, Vinokur, & Ng, 1996). Furthermore, others may do and say things that are disruptive rather than helpful (Dakof & Taylor, 1990; Revenson, Wolman, & Felton, 1983).

Emotional support (e.g., listening, empathizing) can be the most beneficial form of support, but it can also be the most harmful if it is mismanaged (Helgeson & Cohen, 1996). This suggests that patients need to communicate clearly and explicitly (i.e., assertively) what they want others to do (and not do). Some evidence suggests that emotional support from people who are experiencing a similar stressor can be more helpful than support from others (Wortman & Lehman, 1985), especially when the support comes from people who seem to be more well adjusted (Stanton, Danoff-Burg, Cameron, Snider, & Kirk, 1999). This suggests the potential importance of teaching patients about assertiveness and other interpersonal skills in the context of a positive, functional supportive group of other patients.

Recent work also suggests that supportive group interventions may provide important opportunities for upward and downward social comparisons. The patients who are able to perceive themselves as most similar to "upward" targets (i.e., the most well adjusted group members) and least similar to "downward" targets (i.e., the most physically ill group members) may gain the most from these types of interventions (Stanton et al., 1999). Finally, researchers now know that the influence of ethnic, spiritual and religious, and cultural factors is likely to play a critical role in the way patients with cancer adjust to their diagnosis and treatment and experience group support and other psychosocial interventions (Alferi, Culver, Carver, Arena, & Antoni, 1999; Meyerowitz, Richardson, Hudson, & Leedham, 1998). Therefore, the most successful psychosocial group interventions are those that incorporate ethnic and cultural considerations into their content and format.

FINDING BENEFICIAL ASPECTS OF THE CANCER EXPERIENCE

Although most of the psycho-oncology research conducted over the past several years has focused on identifying psychosocial predictors of poor adjustment and distress after a breast cancer diagnosis, researchers are becoming more interested in studying factors that may result in psychological improvements during this period. Researchers and clinicians are now aware that being treated for cancer can have sequelae that patients consider positive. Relatively often, patients report such experiences as improvements in personal resources and skills, an enhanced sense of purpose, an enhanced spirituality, closer relationships with significant others, and changes in their life priorities (e.g., Dow, Ferrell, Leigh, Ly, & Gulasekaram, 1996; Ferrell, Dow, Leigh, Ly, & Gulasekaram, 1995; Ferrell,

Grant, Funk, Otis-Green, & Garcia, 1997; Fromm, Andrykowski, & Hunt, 1996; Kahn & Steeves, 1993; Kurtz, Wyatt, & Kurtz, 1995). Such findings among patients with cancer join a growing literature suggesting that traumatic events can have positive results (e.g., Affleck & Tennen, 1996; Aldwin, Sutton, & Lachman, 1996; Ebersole & Flores, 1989; Lehman et al., 1993; McMillen, Smith, & Fisher, 1997; McMillen, Zuravin, & Rideout, 1995; O'Leary & Ickovics, 1995; Park, Cohen, & Murch, 1996; Schaefer & Moos, 1992; Tedeschi & Calhoun, 1995, 1996). It appears that finding benefits in trauma decreases distress later (McMillen et al., 1997), possibly by permitting resolution of the experience and allowing people to move on with their lives (Carver & Scheier, 1998).

Positive sequelae of traumas come in many forms. Confronting a life-threatening disease may change one's attitude toward life (e.g., by changing priorities and promoting a clearer sense of purpose in life), enhance interpersonal relationships, promote positive health behavior changes (e.g., taking a more active role in maintaining one's own health), and foster a sense of restful repose and focused attention. These positive sequelae are collectively referred to as *positive states of mind* (Adler, Horowitz, Garcia, & Moyer, 1998). Maintaining optimism may be relevant to this experience (Affleck & Tennen, 1996).

Tedeschi and Calhoun (1995) have also suggested that clinical intervention can help foster growth after major stressors or trauma. Our work suggests that this may indeed be the case for women with breast cancer who participate in time-limited, group-based cognitive–behavioral stress management (CBSM) interventions (Antoni et al., 2001). We tested the effects of a 10-week group-based CBSM intervention among 100 women who had recently been treated for stage I or II breast cancer. The intervention reduced prevalence of moderate depression (which remained relatively stable in the control group) but did not affect other measures of emotional distress. The intervention also resulted in more women stating that breast cancer had made positive contributions to their lives; it also increased generalized optimism. Both of these results remained at the 3-month and 9-month follow-ups after the intervention. Additional analyses revealed that the intervention had its greatest impact on generalized optimism among women who at baseline were the least optimistic.

Psychosocial Factors: The Course of Breast Cancer

Solid evidence shows that women with breast cancer experience many concerns during the period of surgery and adjuvant therapy. In addition, personality (e.g., intrapsychic) and contextual (e.g., interpersonal) factors may predict optimal psychosocial adjustment in patients with breast cancer during this period. It follows that psychosocial interventions teaching new cognitive strategies (e.g., cognitive restructuring, coping-skills training) and interpersonal skills (e.g., assertion training, anger management) in the context of a supportive group environment may significantly improve a woman's adjustment to breast cancer and its treatment. It also seems that such adjustment may go far beyond the reduction of acute distress levels; it may actually involve a psychological growth process involving a new sense of meaning and other long-lasting benefits.

Does any evidence show that making such psychological changes during the cancer experience might affect a woman's physical health? Could these psychosocial factors contribute to the actual course of the cancer?

A wide range of psychosocial factors have been associated with the course of established cancer, although the research is replete with inconsistencies (Fox, 1998; Helgeson, Cohen, & Fritz, 1998). These inconsistencies may be a result of the heterogeneity in the samples of patients studied (e.g., mixed cancer types and stages); psychosocial variables assessed; psychosocial interventions used; and the study designs, control variables, and analytic procedures used to establish treatment efficacy. Several authors (Andersen, Kiecolt-Glaser, & Glaser, 1994; Antoni & Goodkin, 1996; Cohen & Rabin, 1998; van der Pompe et al., 1994) have proposed that psychosocial factors may relate more reliably to health outcomes in cancers that are at their earlier stages and are controlled to some degree by immunological or endocrine processes known to be associated with psychosocial factors.

Some of the cancers whose progression seems to be associated with psychosocial factors on the one hand and immune or endocrine system components on the other include malignant melanoma (Fonteneau et al., 1997); breast cancer (J. Miller et al., 1997); prostate cancer (Hwang, Fein, Levitsky, & Nelson, 1999; Stone, Mezzacappa, Brooke, & Gonder, 1999); and virus-related cancers such as cervical cancer (Clerici, Shearer, & Clerici, 1998; Stanley, 1997), and Burkitt's lymphoma, Kaposi's sarcoma, and hepatocellular carcinomas (Bovbjerg & Valdimarsdottir, 1998). Psychosocial factors such as active coping have been shown to predict greater survival time (Fawzy et al., 1993), whereas repressive coping predicts shorter survival in patients with malignant melanoma (Rogentine et al., 1979). In one study, patients with melanoma who had died or whose disease had progressed were matched according to demographic and medical characteristics with patients who had no evidence of disease at the follow-up assessment. Patients who had an unfavorable outcome (e.g., who died or whose disease progressed) had reported greater dysphoric mood and distress 1 to 3 years previously. Overall, these findings suggest that psychosocial factors such as mood may relate to disease progression in patients with melanoma.

Have similar psychosocial factors been associated with the course of breast cancer? Patients with breast cancer experiencing numerous life stressors may be at risk for a relapse or shortened survival time after treatment (Ramirez et al., 1989), although other work refutes this theory (Barraclough et al., 1992). Poor expression of anger (Pettingale, Morris, Greer, & Haybittle, 1985), stoicism (Greer, 1991), repression (Jensen, 1987), and lack of social support (Levy, Herberman, Lippman, & d'Angelo, 1987) all have been related to poorer prognosis in patients with breast cancer as well. Elevated stress levels after adjuvant therapy predicted shorter time to recurrence in patients with breast cancer (Levy, Herberman, Lippman, d'Angelo, & Lee, 1991). Some work suggests that the ways patients with breast cancer react to the stress of diagnosis (e.g., general distress, depression, maintenance of a "fighting spirit") may also predict the course of disease (e.g., Greer, Morris, & Pettingale, 1979; Greer, Morris, Pettingale, & Haybittle, 1990), although other researchers did not find a link between depression and cancer prognosis (Barraclough et al., 1992; Jamison et al., 1978). It seems likely that the discrepancies among these studies stem from methodological differences (N. Mulder, Pompe, Speigel, Antoni, & Vries, 1992; Watson & Ramirez, 1991). For instance, in studies that rely on individuals' self-reports of their attitude after they receive a cancer diagnosis, it is entirely possible that their attitude is highly colored by the severity of their diagnosis, a factor that is usually highly predictive of disease outcomes. The best studies are those that collect psychological information before a diagnosis has been made.

One study found that helplessness and hopelessness responses made before the diagnostic workup are also predictive of disease course (Greer, 1991). A more recent study from this group reported that among 578 women with breast cancer, an increased risk of relapse or death during a 5-year period was associated with elevated scores on helplessness and hopelessness attitudes on the Mental Adjustment to Cancer Scale but was unrelated to stoicism, denial, or fighting spirit (Watson et al., 1999). Importantly, these attitudes may be modifiable by cognitive therapy in patients with breast cancer (Greer et al., 1992). The latter suggests that psychosocial intervention may affect mental and possibly physical health outcomes in patients with breast cancer.

Some key questions are now emerging in the field of psycho-oncology: *What are the consistent psychosocial predictors of cancer disease progression, and what are their likely mediators and effects sizes? How can these associations be used to inform psychosocial interventions?*

Despite numerous inconsistencies in previous research, more recent work relating psychosocial factors to cancer recurrence and survival has produced some interesting results that relate to breast cancer. To clarify the mechanisms underlying these relationships, newer research explores the degree to which psychosocial factors such as stress, social support, coping strategies, and emotional expression relate to physiological regulatory processes (e.g., endocrine and immune systems) that could control the rate of progression and course of the cancer. Understanding the relevance of these phenomena to cancer in psycho-oncology research requires a review of some critical biological factors in breast cancer research (information that is summarized in the next section). The discussion then moves on to the interface among psychosocial factors, the endocrine and immune systems, and cancer.

Biological Factors: The Course of Breast Cancer

Health psychologists who study the association among psychological factors, biological processes, and the course of breast cancer often focus on at least one biological system (e.g., the immune system, the endocrine system) that has previously been related to psychological phenomena such as stress, depression, or other distress states. However, psychologists focusing on this aspect of research should be aware that the links among some of these biological systems and the course of breast cancer have not yet been worked out. For instance, basic questions concerning the role of the immune system in the onset and spread of cancer are still occupying the minds of countless scientists in labs across the world. Just what do we know?

THE ROLE OF THE IMMUNE SYSTEM IN CANCER INITIATION AND PROMOTION

The role of the immune system in the initiation, promotion, and recurrence of different types of carcinomas in humans is an area of continuing debate (Bovbjerg, 1991; Bovbjerg & Valdimarsdottir, 1996; Cohen & Rabin, 1998). At least two major considerations exist regarding the ways in which the status of an individual's immune system might affect the course of cancer-related disease processes. One consideration concerns the role of the immune system in the initiation and promotion of the neoplastic disease process in a person who is at risk for cancer. Another concerns the role of the immune system in the recurrence (and metastases) of cancer in an individual who has been provided with curative and adjuvant treatments. Certain aspects of the immune system are particularly well suited to respond to the initiation or recurrence of tumor growth, some of which include measures that have been previously associated with stressors and other psychosocial factors. However, other tumor-relevant immunological measures have not been well studied by psycho-oncology investigators.

Cells of the Immune System

Neoplastically transformed cells may be destroyed by highly evolved antibodies (chemical neutralizers) made by *B lymphocytes* and can be killed directly by *cytotoxic (killer) T lymphocytes* (CTLs). More primitive and less specific methods involve *macrophages* (the cells of the immune system) and *natural killer (NK) cells* (Brittenden, Heys, Ross, & Eremin, 1996; Cerottini, Lienard, & Romero, 1996; Greenberg & Riddell, 1992). The macrophage is a class of cell usually associated with antigen presentation and processing and phagocytic activity. Activated macrophages have been shown in vitro (in laboratory cultures) to kill various tumor cells including breast cancer cells. A summary of these cells and some of their associated functions is included in Table 1.1.

The cells of the immune system rarely work in isolation. For instance, eradication of tumors in vivo (inside the tumor-bearing host) can involve T-lymphocyte-mediated macrophage killer activity that is initiated by a substance called *interferon-gamma* (IFN-γ). This is but one example of the ways in which different immune cells (e.g., T lymphocytes, macrophages) can work together to attack cancer cells. When people think about an immune response to a tumor, they often think of one of the immune system's killer mechanisms that has evolved for dealing with anomalies such as virus-transformed and cancerous cells. Following is a discussion of some of these mechanisms.

Cancer-Killing Mechanisms

A key killer mechanism, *antibody-dependent cellular cytotoxicity* (ADCC), involves the binding of tumor-specific antibodies to the surface of tumor cells. The antibodies interact with other cells using specialized *Fc receptors,* and the tumor cells are subsequently destroyed from the outside to the inside by soluble chemical mediators. Although the importance of this mechanism for the destruction of tumors in vivo is still not clear, ADCC has been shown to decrease with progression of some cancers (Satam, Suraiya, & Nadkarni, 1986). Cytotoxic (killer) functions can occur through several additional mechanisms. Another cytotoxic function, *natural killer cell cytotoxicity* (NKCC), does not require binding to an antigen-specific receptor. Because of this flexibility, NK cells may represent a first line of defense against the growth of newly transformed cells at primary and metastatic sites, as has been demonstrated for both breast (Levy,

TABLE 1.1

Immune System Cells, Functions, and Chemical Messengers Involved in Defense Against Cancer

Name	Abbreviation or alternate name	Definition
Cells		
CD4+ T lymphocytes	CD4+ cells	"Helper" lymphocytes that coordinate immune cell growth and killer functions
CD8+ T lymphocytes	Cytotoxic T lymphocytes (CTLs)	CTLs that attach to and kill cancerous cells
CD56+ lymphocytes	Natural killer (NK) cells	NK cells that attach to and kill cancerous cells
Macrophages	—	Primitive monocytes that engulf debris but which can be induced to kill tumors
Dendritic cells	DCs	Monocytes that detect, carry, and present parts of cancerous cells to lymphocytes to begin the killing process
Functions		
Lymphocyte proliferative response	LPR	Process by which primed lymphocytes clone to form an army of like-minded cells
Natural killer cell cytotoxicity	NKCC	Process by which NK cells kill tumor-transformed and virally transformed host cells
CTL-mediated cellular cytotoxicity	CTL killing	Process by which CTLs kill tumor-transformed and virally transformed host cells
Antibody-dependent cellular cytotoxicity	ADCC	CTL or NK killing that requires attachment of an antibody to the surface of the cancerous cell
Chemical messengers (cytokines)		
Interleukin-2	IL-2	Promotes lymphocyte proliferative response
Interleukin-4	IL-4	Promotes antibody production from B lymphocytes
Interleukin-10	IL-10	Promotes antibody differentiation in B lymphocytes; blocks IL-2 actions
Interleukin-12	IL-12	Promotes the killing actions of NK cells
Interferon-gamma	IFN-γ	Promotes the killing actions of a wide range of cells including CTLs, NK cells, and macrophages
Tumor necrosis factor	TNF	Interferes directly with actions of tumor cells

Herberman, Lippman, & d'Angelo, 1987; Levy, Herberman, Maluish, Schlein, & Lippman, 1985; Levy, Herberman, & Whiteside, 1990) and cervical carcinomas (Pillai, Balaram, Abraham, Padmanabhan, & Nair 1988; Tay, Jenkins, & Singer, 1987). A third mechanism, *CTL-mediated immunity*, may also play a role in the recognition and destruction of tumor cells, especially of virus-initiated cancers such as cervical cancer and some of the lymphomas (Melief, 1992). Finally, it is known that *helper T cells* (CD4+ cells), although not specifically killer cells, can be critical in orchestrating the production of chemical messengers by CTLs, NK cells, and macrophages. *Just how do these messengers work?*

One chemical component of the immune system relevant to tumor initiation and promotion is a set of substances often referred to as the *soluble mediators* of the immune system—the *cytokines*. Many cytokines are associated with coordinating immunological defenses against tumors— cytokines such as *tumor necrosis factor-beta* (TNF-β), which can have direct suppressive effects on tumors themselves, and *interleukin-2* (IL-2), which is used to produce *lymphokine-activated killer cells* (LAK cells), which resemble NK cells in many ways and are used as a cancer treatment technique. Finally, IFN-γ has both direct toxic effects on cancer cells and immune-boosting effects through NKCC. Emerging work has focused on the use of other cytokines such as IL-12, which has potent effects on NKCC, possibly by priming T-cell production of IFN-γ (Gerosa et al., 1996).

Note that some cytokines, such as IL-4 and IL-10, lack antitumor properties and may actually work against some of the substances just listed. This "yin-yang" model has prompted immunological researchers to classify cytokines made by T helper cells (the primary orchestrators of the immune system) as those that promote functions such cell-mediated cytotoxicity (killing) and those that are involved in humoral activities affecting inflammation. Within the context of cancer-fighting actions, cytokines such as IL-2, IL-12, and IFN-γ that are associated with killing functions are referred to as *T-helper-type 1* (Th1) cells. Those more associated with humoral functions, such as IL-4 and IL-10, are referred to as *T-helper-type 2* (Th2) cytokines. Some work suggests that the ratio of Th1:Th2 cytokines may play a key role in the promotion and progression of breast cancer and cervical cancer (Clerici et al., 1997; Gruijl et al., 1999; Tsukui et al., 1996).

For the purposes of this book and psycho-oncology research per se, it is important to note that emerging evidence now shows that several of these immunological factors and processes, including the T-helper cells, CTLs, and NK cells and processes such as NKCC and Th1 and Th2 cytokine production, may be influenced by psychosocial factors such as stressors, depression, and stress management interventions (Antoni, Cruess, Wagner, et al., 2000; Herbert & Cohen, 1993a, 1993b).

What else in the immune system could influence the course of a cell that has become cancerous? The next section introduces some newer ideas emerging from the fields of tumor biology and tumor immunology that may in the next few years become targeted areas of investigation for health psychologists studying patients with cancer.

Deactivating Damaged or Cancerous Cells: Programmed Cell Death

In addition to the role of specific immunological factors in monitoring and eradicating neoplastic development, the immune system's role in the destruction or repair of damaged DNA may have direct consequences on cancer incidence. Once a cell is beyond the point of repair, *apoptosis*, or programmed cell death, is initiated. Apoptosis can occur through one of three mechanisms: (a) *genetic apoptosis* via the *p53* gene, a cancer gene associated with repression or suppression of cancerous cells; (b) *tumor-initiated apoptosis*, which involves "death signals" sent from cancer cells through FAS ligands to receiving points (FAS receptors) on T lympho-cytes; and (c) *immunologically initiated apoptosis*, which involves proteolytic enzymes such as granzymes that are produced by cells such as CTLs and NK cells (Israels & Israels, 1999). Apoptosis is a normal physiological pro-cess through which aberrant cells (i.e., tumor cells) are cleared from the body. Interactions on the cell membranes or within the cells trigger a cascade of mechanisms leading to cell death (Finkel, 1999; Tomei et al., 1990; Trauth et al., 1989). Numerous carcinogens can damage the DNA of host cells (e.g., ultraviolet radiation from sunlight that can result in malignant melanoma). A failure to repair or destroy these cells could leave the host vulnerable to the proliferation of mutant cells, thereby increasing the likelihood of cancer. Some data have suggested that even moderate psychosocial stressors can compromise the DNA repair process (Glaser, Thorn, Tarr, Kiecolt-Glaser, & D'Ambrosio, 1985).

How Cancerous Cells Escape the Body's Immune Defenses

Another strategy for studying the associations between host defense mechanisms and cancer outcomes involves investigations of a phenom-enon called *immunological escape*. Despite the impressive collection of an-titumor defenses, tumors have many ways to elude the immune system and become clinically evident cancer (Melief, 1992). Cancer cells can lose their surface antigens, thus fooling the immune system into think-ing they are normal cells (Ljunggren & Karre, 1990). They can also mask their surface with large molecules, such as the mucin called *MUC-1* that plays an important role in breast cancer (Seymour, Pettit, O'Flaherty, Charnley, & Kirby, 1999; Zhang, Sikut, & Hansson, 1997). The cells may also suppress CTLs, which short-circuits an important cancer-cell-killing mechanism (Awwad & North, 1990). Finally, some cancerous cells are able to express regulatory proteins (e.g., Bcl-2) that inhibit tumor cell apoptosis (Aizawa et al., 1999).

An emerging area of science involves investigations of tumor-secreted agents, such as *transforming growth factor-beta* (TGF-β) and *vascular endo-*

thelial growth factor (VEGF), that promote activities needed for tumor growth such as the formation of new blood vessels, or *angiogenesis*, and inhibit activities needed for cancer control such as the clonal expansion of T lymphocytes that recognize the tumor cells as foreign, the induction of CTLs, and the maturation of specialized recognition cells called *dendritic cells* (Gabrilovich et al., 1996). Growing evidence suggests that the cancer process itself can disturb apoptosis in those with breast cancer (Reed, 1999) or prostate cancer (Bruckheimer, Gjertsen, & McDonnell, 1999; LaCasse, Baird, Korneluk, & MacKenzie, 1998).

Very little is currently known about the way psychosocial factors might contribute to or hinder immunological escape. Most of the biological processes reviewed so far have been suggested to be more or less relevant for the initiation and early promotion of cancerous cell changes. The general idea is that people are equipped with defenses that may halt precancerous or neoplastic cell changes before they develop into clinically manifest and diagnosable cancer. Later in this book is an introduction to what is known about the associations among some of the biological processes and psychosocial factors relevant to stress management. However, it is important to understand that some additional biological processes may be more relevant to controlling cancerous growth once it has already become clinically manifest. Once a cancer is diagnosed, a person's primary tumor may continue to grow locally, begin to spread from the primary site to surrounding tissues, recur at a new site once it has been surgically removed, or all of these. Following is a review of some of the immunological processes that may be relevant for managing some of these cancer-related activities. It is these interactions that may determine the actual course of the disease, the physical health of the host, and the changes in quality of life that a patient with a condition such as breast cancer may experience over time.

The Immunological Repertoire: Preventing Cancer Progression and Recurrence

Once a cancerous process has been established and diagnosed, it is common that an individual will undergo "curative" treatments such as surgery and lymph node removal. However, in numerous cases, the initial cancerous process continues to develop; the tumor cells may spread to distant body sites, resulting in a relapse, or *recurrence*, of the disease years later. Much research has been dedicated to studying which immunological factors are best equipped to monitor and arrest such continued growth and spread of disease. The NK cells and CTLs are believed to play an important role in the host response against circulating tumor cells in the early stages of disease, and perhaps those spread mechanically during surgery, thus preventing metastases (Gorelik & Herberman, 1989; Melief & Kast, 1991; Trinchieri, 1989).

Among patients with solid tumors, greater NKCC predicted longer survival time without metastases during a 13-year period (Pross & Baines, 1988). Lower NKCC also predicted development of local recurrence of colorectal cancer (Brittenden et al., 1996) and distant metastases in patients with head and neck tumors (Schantz & Goephert, 1987). Patients with breast cancer have been shown to display significantly lower NKCC, even those in stages I to III (Shevde, Joshi, Dudhat, Hawaldar, & Nadkarni, 1999), and NKCC seems to be even lower in patients in stage IV (Baxevanis et al., 1993; Konjevic & Spuzic, 1992, 1993) and in those with liver metastases (Yamasaki et al., 1993).

Interestingly, patients with breast cancer with *estrogen-receptor* positive (ER+) tumors have greater T-cell numbers and cytolytic immune function than those with ER– tumors, suggesting a possible immune mechanism underlying the well-known better prognosis for patients with ER+ tumors (Shevde et al., 1999). As breast cancer progresses from stage II to IV, T-lymphocyte numbers and function become significantly reduced (Contreras Ortiz & Stoliar, 1988). Patients with breast cancer also have lower total T-cell counts and lymphocyte proliferative responses to challenge (Shevde et al., 1999). Patients with lower T-lymphocyte counts and lymphocyte proliferation before surgery have a higher risk for recurrent disease (Hacene et al., 1986; Wiltschke et al., 1995).

Two other cells often associated with innate or natural immunity— dendritic cells and macrophages—are believed to be important in the course of some cancers. Dendritic cells play a key role in tumor antigen presentation, are potent stimulators of T cells (Grabbe, Beissert, Schwarz, & Granstein, 1995; Mayordomo et al., 1995), and have been associated with longer survival in patients with cancer (Ishigami et al., 1998). It is now known that macrophages stimulated with certain cytokines can kill tumor cells (Greenberg, 1991). It is important to note that macrophages have also been implicated in the aberrant induction of apoptosis of viable T cells and NK cells in the local environment of tumors, suggesting that they may work against other tumor-fighting immune cells (Kiessling et al., 1999).

Using the Immune System as a Form of Breast Cancer Therapy

The past decade has included significant work in immunotherapy with cytokines known as *biological response modifiers*. Such research includes the Th1 cytokines IL-2 and IFN-γ and their role in the treatment of different cancers including breast cancer and malignant melanoma (DeVita, Hellman, & Rosenberg, 1997). The previously mentioned LAK cells, which are NK-like cells that have been stimulated with substances such as IL-2 or IFN-γ to become killers, may be more cytotoxic than resting NK cells and be effective against a wider variety of tumor cells, including breast cancer cells (Baxevanis et al., 1993; Whiteside & Herberman, 1990). Other work has shown that patients with liver metastases from breast cancer had increases in lymphocyte proliferative responses to IL-2 and autologous tumor extract antigen in mixed culture (IL-2-enhanced mixed lymphocyte tumor response) after adoptive cell transfer, and these increases correlated with survival after treatment (Yamasaki et al., 1993). Lymphocyte count and proliferation rate of cultured lymphocytes were also significantly associated with prognosis (Yamasaki et al., 1993).

A good deal of evidence now suggests the mechanisms by which IL-2 and other cytokines could coordinate the immunological repertoire against breast cancer. In vitro treatment of peripheral blood leukocytes with IL-2 in patients with stages I, II, or III breast cancer provided a dose-dependent enhancement of their NKCC to levels higher than those of healthy controls (Konjevic & Spuzic, 1993). Low-dose subcutaneous IL-2-based immunotherapy significantly increased NK cells and NK/LAK-mediated killing of the MCF-7 breast cell line antigen in patients with breast cancer after autologous transplantation. This suggests that IL-2 stimulation may be an important *in vivo* phenomenon for conferring immunological surveillance in patients with breast cancer and may do so by selectively increasing specific subpopulations of NK cells (J. Miller et al., 1997).

Vaccines Against Cancer?

One very exciting new treatment approach that attempts to use the immune system to treat cancer involves the development of tumor vaccines (Hwang et al., 1999; Weber, 2000) and carcinogenic virus vaccines (e.g., Hines, Ghim, & Jenson, 1996). Vaccines may offer protection against cancer development, progression, and recurrence. The vaccines usually involve combining allogenic or autologous cell lines with substances that increase either antigenicity (e.g., Bacille Calmette-Guerin [BCG]) or cytokines such as IL-2, IL-4, IL-12, or *granulocyte-macrophage–colony-stimulating factors* (GM–CSF), with the latter being the most promising. The immunogenicity of tumor vaccines may also be enhanced by inducing tumor cells to express genes for cytokines such as GM–CSF, IL-2, or IFN-γ (e.g., J. W. Simons et al., 1997). Some of these combination vaccine treatments have shown encouraging results in patients with malignant melanoma (Dranoff et al., 1997). Vaccines developed from tumor differentiation antigens (e.g., MART-1) have also been successful, especially in combination with GM–CSF in the treatment of patients with melanoma.

An emerging branch of tumor vaccine research concerns work designed to stimulate the production of antigen-presenting dendritic cells from the mononuclear cell population using cytokines such as GM-CSF (Roth et al., 2000). One of the major challenges in cancer treatment has been the relatively small numbers of dendritic cells available for antitumor functions, which is partly a result of the ability of certain tumors to induce dendritic cell apoptosis (Esche et al., 1999). When successful, this treatment allows one to use the immune system to fight cancer cells because dendritic cells are the most potent stimulators of naïve and memory T cells. Equally significant is the fact that this treatment has been designed to allow patients to inject themselves with daily doses of these cytokines at home. Because it is known that stressors and certain coping strategies may reduce patients' ability to carry out health care treatments outside of the hospital, it may be important to explore how behavioral interventions can be used to maximize the effectiveness of this line of immunological treatment in patients with breast cancer.

ENDOCRINE FACTORS AND CANCER INITIATION AND PROMOTION

Endocrine (hormonal) factors may play an even more important role than the immune system in the initiation and promotion of breast cancer. The chief sex hormones, also known as *hypothalamic–pituitary–gonadal (HPG)–related hormones*, that have been associated with human cancers are testosterone (for prostate cancer and breast cancer) and estrogens (for breast cancer; Key, 1995). Sound evidence from animal and human studies shows that hormones such as estrogen, progesterone, and prolactin may contribute to the development of breast cancer (see van der Pompe et al., 1994, for review). Recent work suggests that both estradiol and testosterone are associated with an elevated risk for breast cancer (Cauley et al., 1999). Although endogenous estrogens are associated with the growth of extant breast tumors (Key, 1995; van der Pompe et al., 1994), it is known that antiestrogen agents such as tamoxifen may be efficacious in reducing the risk of invasive and noninvasive breast cancer by 50% (Fisher et al., 1998). Thus, it may be that a normalization of HPG levels is a key to maintaining health in women who have developed or are at risk for breast cancer.

Psychoneuroimmunology and Psycho-Oncology

ASSOCIATIONS BETWEEN PSYCHOSOCIAL VARIABLES AND IMMUNE RESPONSES

Several psychosocial variables have been associated with immune system factors that may be relevant to human cancers such as breast cancer.

Stress Hormones and Cancer

Much work has also explored the role of the stress hormones in the mediation of links between stress and cancer. Psychological stressors and stress responses are associated with changes in hypothalamic–pituitary–adreno–cortical hormones, such as cortisol and sympathetic nervous system hormones such as epinephrine (adrenaline) and norepinephrine (noradrenaline), which are in turn associated with decrements in immune system functioning. In fact, much of the theory underlying the subdiscipline of psychoneuroimmunology rests on the assumption that these agents are the communication channel between psychological stress experiences and immune system changes. What remains to be determined is whether these proposed mechanisms can be used to explain the association between similar psychological phenomena and cancer-related processes (i.e., initiation, progression, recurrence). Some of this research is explained in the context of breast cancer in a later section of this chapter.

Some of these immune responses include the T-lymphocyte response, some of which (CTLs) have the potential to kill cancerous cells; lymphocyte proliferative responses to challenge (an index of the immune system's ability to clonally expand in response to antigens); and NK cells and their ability to kill tumor targets in vitro (NKCC). Higher levels of each of these immune responses are believed to afford individuals with greater protection from or surveillance over cancerous cells, so health psychologists often examine how psychological phenomena such as stress relate to decrements in these immune system parameters, possibly causing poorer health outcomes in patients dealing with cancer or patients who are at a higher risk for developing cancer.

For instance, poorer social support (Levy et al., 1991) and greater distress levels (Andersen et al., 1998) have been related to decrements in NKCC among patients with early-stage breast cancer. Patients with early-stage breast cancer who had greater distress after surgery had lower NKCC by 15 months after surgery; lower NKCC at this time point predicted a shorter time to recurrence in the 5- to 8-year follow-up (Levy et al., 1990). Growing evidence suggests that stressors and distress states are related to poorer NKCC and lymphocyte proliferation in patients with breast cancer at varying stages of disease and treatment (Andersen et al., 1998; Bovbjerg & Valdimarsdottir, 1993; van der Pompe et al., 1994). However, there still remains a disconnect between studies relating stress and psychosocial factors to immune status and those relating the same psychosocial factors to disease relapse and survival in patients with cancer.

One burning question remains in psycho-oncology research: *Do the ways that people respond to stressors (i.e., their distress states and depressive symptoms, their coping strategies, their use of social support) relate to changes in NKCC, which in turn predicts disease-free intervals and survival time among patients with cancer?* Without such evidence, it remains unclear whether the associations between psychosocial factors and disease course are mediated by *affective–psychoneuroimmunological mechanisms*. In other words this suggests that active coping effects on distress reduction may be accompanied by reductions in immunosuppressive stress hormones such as cortisol. Alternatively, this association could be explained using *health behavior mechanisms*. For example, people using more active coping and social isolation are more conscientious about follow-up medical care and reducing their exposure to risk factors. Unfortunately, previous studies showing the health benefits of psychosocial interventions for patients with breast cancer did not provide definitive evidence for either of these possible paths (e.g., Spiegel, Bloom, Kraemer, & Gottheil, 1989). Without such information, it is impossible to isolate mechanisms explaining the health effects of these sorts of interventions. It is likely that the effects involve a bit of each pathway and that the combined effect of both is still much less than the influence of genetic factors and ongoing treatments.

For the purposes of this book, a model is included that suggests some of the ways that psychosocial factors such as cognitive coping strategies, self-efficacy, and social support might explain individual differences in the reactions of patients to the stress of having cancer (see Figure 1.1). We propose that these psychological reactions may be accompanied by changes in stress hormones (e.g., dysregulation of catecholamine and cortisol production) and sex hormones (e.g., increased testosterone) that may relate directly or indirectly to disease recurrence by their suppressive effects on different aspects of the immunological response to cancer. We also propose that these psychological reactions may relate to disease course through their effects on positive and negative health behaviors, which may or may not involve these biological pathways. For instance, a woman who is depressed and is dealing with breast cancer may fail to follow up after her surgery, may refrain from seeking out important information about newly emerging treatments, or may not be motivated to make lifestyle changes that are necessary for optimizing health outcomes. Numerous theoretical models such as these have been proposed for health psychology researchers working with patients with different types of cancer (e.g., Andersen et al., 1994).

FIGURE 1.1

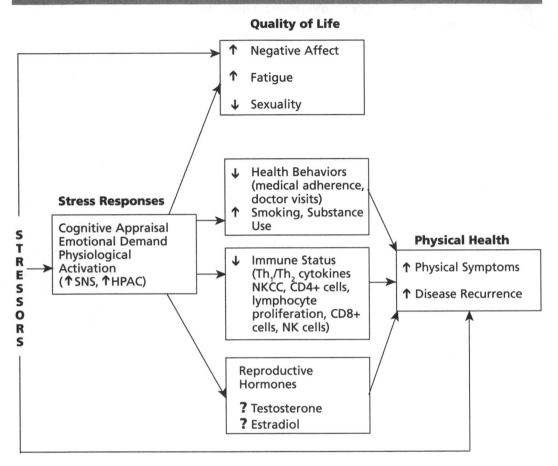

PSYCHOSOCIAL FACTORS AND IMMUNE RESPONSE ASSOCIATIONS IN PATIENTS WITH BREAST CANCER

In various populations, psychosocial factors (stressors, distress states, pessimism, poor social support) and lifestyle behavioral variables (e.g., smoking) have been associated with changes in cell counts and percentages of lymphocytes known to be relevant to promotion of some types of cancer, including cervical and breast cancers (e.g., NK and CTL cell counts, NKCC; Byrnes et al., 1998; Goodkin, Blaney, Feaster, & Fletcher, 1992; Irwin, Daniels, Smith, Bloom, & Weiner, 1987; Kiecolt-Glaser et al., 1986; Levy et al., 1987). Behavioral scientists are now conducting prospective studies to determine whether one can predict disease progression and survival on the basis of these psychoimmune associations in patients who have been diagnosed with breast cancer. However, it is now becoming apparent that the strength of these associations may vary as a function of the patient's age, stage of disease, and personal cancer history.

PERSONAL HISTORY OR FAMILY HISTORY OF CANCER

One research group found that having a cancer history actually moderated the association between stressors and NKCC, so that only those with a prior history of cancer demonstrated the hypothesized negative correlation between life hassles and NKCC (Vitaliano et al., 1998). Patients with a familial history of melanoma have lower NKCC (Hersey, Edwards, Honeyman, & McCarthy, 1979), and genetic studies suggest that this may be a result of deficits in IL-12 receptor expression (Altare et al., 1998). This is important when one considers that once diagnosed and treated for malignant melanoma, patients with greater NKCC in the months after surgery show greater survival in the 6 following years (Fawzy et al., 1993). Another group found that women at familial risk for breast cancer had significant associations between heightened emotional distress and decreased NKCC (Bovbjerg & Valdimarsdottir, 1993). This work suggests the intriguing possibility that psychosocial factors in certain individuals who are less able to manage stressors may actually interact with genetic factors to create a "vulnerability" for greater immune system decrements and increased cancer risk. These investigators have proposed that future psycho-oncology researchers should examine the association between familial history of cancer and a wide range of psychosocial behavioral factors that may influence cancer outcomes through the immune system (Bovbjerg & Valdimarsdottir, 1996). Therefore, it seems plausible that men and women with predisposing genetic, psychosocial, and lifestyle factors for the development of cancer (e.g., women with a *BRCA* gene) may be especially good candidates for psychosocial interventions hypothesized to modulate stress-sensitive immune functions such as NKCC.

PSYCHOSOCIAL–ENDOCRINE–IMMUNE MECHANISMS IN PATIENTS WITH CANCER

Because psychosocial interventions may affect patients with cancer by modulating perceived stressors, stress responses, and emotional expressivity, understanding the role of stress-associated neuroendocrine substances and their regulation is important. To the extent that changes in these hormones are associated directly through tumor initiation and promotion or indirectly through impairments in immune surveillance and DNA repair abilities, they are important to study as possible mediators of psychosocial influences on the course of human cancers such as breast cancer.

One of the most commonly cited explanations for stress and immunity associations concerns the endocrine changes that are believed to occur during and after one's appraisals of and coping responses to stressor events (Antoni, 1997). An individual's perception of the availability of a coping response in a stressful situation has been shown to trigger a series of physiological events that lead to specific neurological, endocrine, and immunological responses (McEwen, 1998). The neuroendocrine mediation of immune suppression involves two major systems—the *hypothalamic–pituitary–adrenocortical system* (HPAC) and the *sympathetic adrenomedullary system* (SAM)—the systems controlling the secretion of the stress hormones. A specific pattern of acute nervous system activity coordinated by the HPAC and SAM systems occurs when coping responses to stressors are available. This pattern is referred to as *active coping*, or the *fight-or-flight* response. Activation of the SAM system involves release of neurohormones called *catecholamines*—specifically norepinephrine and epinephrine—into the circulation, which prepares a person to physically confront or flee from the stressor. Another physiological response pattern occurs when coping responses are not available. This behavioral pattern is known as *passive coping*, or *conservation–withdrawal*, and is accompanied by hypervigilance without movement. This response is elicited by ambiguous, unpredictable, and uncontrollable situations and is generally associated with persistent, repeated, and chronic HPAC activation (Antoni, 1987; Mason, 1975; McCabe & Schneiderman, 1985). The HPAC activation and lack of homeostatic adjustment may increase the secretion of *hypothalamic corticotropin-releasing hormone* (CRH), possibly resulting in increased secretion of *adrenocorticotrophic hormone* (ACTH) from the pituitary gland and increased release of cortisol from the adrenal cortex. Cortisol has been shown to suppress numerous components of the immune system that may affect cancer processes (Maier, Watkins, & Fleshner, 1994).

Activation of the SAM and HPAC systems, systems that interact with one another (Axelrod & Reisine, 1984), adversely affects immunological status (Crary et al., 1983; Cupps & Fauci, 1982; Roszman & Brooks, 1985). These changes may be especially important in view of the notion that some cancers secrete agents such as CRH and ACTH, which can modulate the HPAC system, thereby maintaining an environment supportive of malignant cell invasion and migration through corticosteroid-induced immunosuppression (Cox & MacKay, 1982). More recently, research with humans has shown that cortisol and catecholamines decrease production of Th1 cytokines such as IFN-γ and IL-12 and increase production of Th2 cytokines such as IL-10 (Agarwal & Marshall, 1998; Elenkov, Papanicolaou, Wilder, & Chrousos, 1996). Note that Th1 cytokines such as

IFN-γ and IL-12 have been shown to be critical for optimal NK-cell-mediated killing of tumor targets. Thus, it seems important that a person have sufficient numbers of killer cells as well as have the killing capacity. The Th1 cytokines seem capable of instilling NK cells with the killing instructions needed to attack and immobilize cancer cells. On the other hand, Th2 cytokines such as IL-10, which are important for inflammatory responses and allergic reactions, may actually interfere with the ability of Th1 cytokines to do their job through a direct antagonistic process. Therefore, shifts toward Th2 cytokine production, which may be instigated by stress hormones such as cortisol, may work toward impairing the ability of Th1 cytokines to signal a strong NKCC response and have been postulated to promote neoplastic processes such as breast cancer (Clerici et al., 1998).

A third possible system involving neuroendocrine mediation of immunological changes triggered by stressors involves opiate peptides. Shavit et al. (1986) provided evidence suggesting that specific opiate receptors in the brain are responsible for morphine-induced suppression of NKCC. Although the underlying physiological mechanism is not yet clearly understood, it is possible that opiate peptides may affect NK cells through their activation of the HPAC system, stimulating the release of cortisol (Shavit et al., 1987).

A fourth type of endocrine-mediated immunological changes is stressor-induced changes in neuroactive hormones released by the lymphocytes themselves, which may be active in the central nervous system (CNS) and the peripheral areas of the nervous system (e.g., spinal ganglia; Blalock, Bost, & Smith, 1985; Besedovsky et al., 1983; G. R. Smith, McKenzie, Marmer, & Steel, 1985).

A fifth possible endocrine-mediated immune mechanism especially relevant for certain cancers involves the effects of HPG hormones such as estrogens, progesterone, and testosterone on the immune system (or as previously noted, directly on tumors; van der Pompe et al., 1994). Estradiol and testosterone administration causes NKCC reductions (Hou & Zheng, 1988), and increases in estrogen during the menstrual cycle (Sulke, Jones, & Wood, 1985) and pregnancy (Pope, 1990) are associated with NKCC decreases. Progesterone seems to suppress NKCC and may additionally suppress NKCC when combined with estrogens (Feinberg, Tan, Gonik, Brath, & Walsh, 1991), which could be caused by down regulation of IFN-γ production.

Of the five mediating mechanisms outlined, one of the most commonly proposed as an explanation for associations between psychosocial factors and cancer outcomes involves the relationship among the HPAC system (e.g., cortisol elevations), immune function, and tumor progression. Twenty years ago, animal studies indicated that the activity of macrophages and NK cells against tumor growth was inhibited by psychosocial-stressor-induced elevations in adrenal corticosteroids (Newberry, Liebelt, & Boyle, 1984; Pavlidis & Chirigos, 1980). Similarly, a series of studies demonstrated that elevated corticosterone (the rodent equivalent of cortisol) concentrations suppressed IFN production, which as noted is important for augmenting and maintaining NKCC (Cox & Mackay, 1982). Conversely, pharmacological agents that acted as corticosteroid inhibitors facilitated resistance to tumor growth in these mice. Although these findings are suggestive, they have been refuted. With regard to tumor progression, negligible differences between stressor-induced neuroendocrine changes and suppression of tumor growth have been noted (Riley, Fitzmaurice, & Spackman, 1981). These inconsistencies may be due to the possibility that the relationships among stressors, immune changes, and tumor promotion vary greatly as a function of the intensity, chronicity, predictability, and controllability of stressors (Sklar & Anisman, 1979).

To explain some of the findings relating psychosocial factors to breast cancer relapse and survival, some researchers have focused on psychoneuroimmunological mechanisms (van der Pompe et al., 1994). However, in general, the insufficient methodological controls of prior research mean that researchers cannot draw firm psychoneuroimmunological conclusions. Psychosocial stressors may relate to the course of breast cancer through sex hormones (e.g., testosterone) and stress hormones (e.g., cortisol) that contribute directly to tumor growth (Forsyth, 1991; Sutherland, 1987).

More recent work has related distress levels, which were possibly reflecting elevated HPAC activity, with immune status in women with breast cancer during the weeks after surgery. Andersen et al. (1998) showed that greater distress (as measured by the Impact of Event Scale; Horowitz, Wilner, & Alvarez, 1979) related to lower NKCC, lower IFN-γ-stimulated NKCC, and lower lymphoproliferative responses to challenge among 116 patients with stage II or stage III breast cancer in the period after surgery but before adjuvant therapy. These findings were the same after controlling for patient age, disease stage, and recovery time since surgery. The authors concluded that the physiological effects of stress-related processes inhibit cellular immune responses that were relevant to cancer prognosis in these women (Andersen et al., 1998). They also noted that longitudinal studies are needed to determine the duration of these effects, their ability to predict health consequences in patients with breast cancer, and their biological and behavioral mechanisms. One possible mechanism may involve stress-associated increases in cortisol.

Numerous research findings suggest that cortisol is related (through the immune system or independent of the immune system) to the course of breast cancer (van der Pompe et al., 1994). Changes in HPAC axis functioning have been reported in women with breast cancer, including changes in the circadian rhythm of cortisol secretion (Touitou, Bogdan, Levi, Benavides, & Auzeby, 1996; Touitou et al., 1995) and elevations in circulating levels of cortisol (Hays & O'Brian, 1989; Read et al., 1983). Other work suggests that patients with breast cancer also have higher resting cortisol levels and abnormal ACTH (a cortisol-signaling peptide) responses to acute laboratory challenge compared with age-matched healthy women (van der Pompe, Antoni, Visser, Heijnen, & deVries, 1996).

Another interesting phenomenon concerns the daily alterations, or diurnal patterns, of cortisol production, which can be monitored through regular collection of saliva samples during daily activities. Normally, the salivary cortisol levels peak on wakening and gradually decline during the afternoon, reaching their low point by nightfall. The more a person produces this reliable decline during the day, the greater their *cortisol secretion slope*. One provocative study found that flattened or abnormal diurnal cortisol slopes predicted lower NK cell counts and shorter survival (in 5 to 6 years) among women with metastatic breast cancer (Sephton, Sapolski, Kraemer, & Spiegel, 2000). Thus, HPAC functioning as a means of explaining relationships between psychosocial factors and the course of breast cancer seems to be an important avenue to explore. If the women's responses to stressors and other life challenges can predict their future psychological adjustment and important physiological changes, they may also affect disease course. It follows that psychological interventions that alter stress responses involving cortisol and other hormones may provide mental and physical health benefits for these women.

Psychosocial Interventions for Patients With Cancer

At least three target areas are relevant to psychosocial intervention research in cancer. The issues involve (a) reducing cancer risk behaviors and improving cancer monitoring behaviors (e.g., use of screening programs and breast self-exams), (b) facilitating psychosocial adjustment to cancer diagnosis and treatment, and (c) optimizing health outcomes and survival after curative treatment efforts. This section focuses on the latter two targets, with attention to studies demonstrating the efficacy of psychosocial interventions. Also included is a summary of the studies exploring the plausible psychosocial and health behavior explanations of these effects, which will help clarify the essential ingredients, optimal timing, and minimum needed length of these interventions, factors that were all taken into consideration in developing and evaluating the B-SMART program.

FACILITATING ADJUSTMENT TO THE CANCER DIAGNOSIS

Individuals who receive a cancer diagnosis are more likely than healthy, disease-free people to be faced with chronic and uncontrollable stressors (e.g., treatment responsiveness and side effects, fears of disease recurrence, changing family roles, waiting for results of additional medical tests, medical costs) as they progress through the uncertain period of cancer treatment. They may also be more prone to lose their familiar sources of social support because of (a) their own desire to withdraw socially in response to changes in physical appearance and increased fatigue and (b) the tendency for acquaintances and significant others to avoid them or "burn out" as their disease progresses. The combination of uncontrollable life stressors and diminishing social resources creates cognitive and emotional burdens that may overwhelm prior, or premorbid, coping strategies (e.g., active coping, making plans), resulting in the use of denial and disengagement strategies and a decreased awareness of and expression of feelings (i.e., emotional numbing). A general sense of the inability to cope may cause decreased self-esteem and self-efficacy, feelings of helplessness and hopelessness, and even symptoms of depression. A decreased sense of self-efficacy is known to decrease effort and perseverance while increasing depression and perceptions of stress (Bandura, 1986). All of these phenomena are salient to an individual coping with breast cancer.

Managing Distress

Members of the medical and oncology community are becoming more aware of the need to create clear guidelines for the management of cancer-related distress (Holland, 2000; Payne, Hoffman, Theodoulou, Dosik, & Massie, 1999; A. Roth et al., 1998; Weber, 2000). Some consider the primary obstacles to appropriate distress management to be (a) the lack of minimum standards for psychosocial care and (b) that many physicians are unaware of ways to obtain this type of care for their patients (Holland, 2000). Other interesting trends likely to affect the care of patients with cancer include a growing respect for the importance of integrating spirituality into the medical arena and the need to improve physician–patient communication (Dolbeault, Szporn, & Holland, 1999; Fallowfield & Jenkins, 1999). For instance, one survey conducted at Memorial Sloan–Kettering Cancer Center found that approximately 75% of patients with cancer believed that religion and spirituality are key coping strategies for dealing with cancer (Holland, 2000).

The National Comprehensive Cancer Network (NCCN), made up of 17 comprehensive cancer centers in the United States, has proposed a psychosocial treatment approach for cancer-related distress that includes appropriate triaging for mental health and pastoral counseling to reduce distress, relieve pain, and meet spiritual needs. They have noted that psychosocial screening should begin in the waiting room at the initial visit, and conditions such as dementia, delirium, anxiety disorder, substance abuse, and personality problems should be grounds for a mental health treatment referral. They recommend that a multidisciplinary committee oversee the guidelines of cancer distress management at each national center. The NCCN report suggests that the benefits of distress management may include better patient–physician communication, enhanced compliance with treatment regimens, and lower mood disturbance and stress.

Importantly, not all patients experience the same difficulties, and they do not experience distress at the same point in the cancer experience. In fact, the emotional issues that patients with cancer encounter seem to be specific to different phases of the disease, changing somewhat from the prediagnostic phase, to the diagnostic phase, to the treatment phase, to the recurrence phase, and (if relevant) to the terminal phase (Fawzy, Fawzy, Hyun, & Wheeler, 1997). During the treatment phase, which is usually initiated by some sort of curative intervention such as surgery, the predominant emotional reactions include feelings of fear and grief. Maladaptive responses might include avoidance, postoperative reactive depression, and a prolonged postoperative grief reaction (Fawzy et al., 1997). However, little psychosocial intervention is offered at this phase. Frequently, only patients with diagnosable depressive or anxiety-related conditions receive mental health treatment, often in the form of a medication prescription.

Education and behavioral training programs are often applied in the earlier phases of disease (the diagnostic and treatment phases), whereas supportive therapy is more common for later phases (the recurrence and terminal phases). The majority of the studies have been conducted with women dealing with breast cancer or groups with a variety of diseases (Fawzy & Fawzy, 1996). The psychosocial interventions developed for patients with cancer to date have usually embodied either a cognitive–behavioral or existential theoretical orientation, which are discussed in the following sections.

COGNITIVE–BEHAVIORAL INTERVENTIONS

Reviews of studies of psychosocial interventions used for patients with cancer (Andersen, 1992; Trijsburg, van Knippenberg, & Rijpma, 1992) have revealed mostly positive effects on indexes of psychosocial adjustment for CBSM. Of the studies reviewed by Trijsburg et al., almost all had stress and distress reduction as the primary goal. Other goals included (in

Intervention Categories

Many psychosocial intervention models have been developed to help patients with cancer deal with the numerous psychological issues that emerge in each phase of the disease experience. The goals of these interventions are to decrease feelings of alienation, reduce anxiety about treatments, clarify misinformation, and decrease feelings of helplessness. Fawzy et al. (1997) noted that these interventions usually fall into one or more of four common categories:

- Education (Brandenburg, Bergenmar, & Bjolund, 1994; Gordon et al., 1980; Richardson, Shelton, Krailo, & Levine, 1990)
- Behavioral training (relaxation and imagery training; Baider, Uziely, & De-Nour, 1994; Bridge, Benson, Pietroni, & Priest, 1998; Gruber et al., 1993)
- Group supportive therapy (Berglund et al., 1994; Greer et al., 1992; Spiegel, Bloom, & Yalom, 1981)
- Individual supportive therapy (Fawzy, 1996; M. Linn, Linn, & Harris, 1982)

descending order) increasing "effective" coping strategies (11 of 22 studies), expression of concerns and feelings (10 studies); preserving social support (9 studies); debunking myths about the illness (8 studies); promoting hope, positive self-image, adequate sexual relations (5 studies); and encouraging relaxation (5 studies). Cognitive–behavioral interventions seem to be the most widely used psychosocial intervention in comprehensive cancer centers in the United States (Coluzzi et al., 1995) and have had a major impact in the areas of pain relief, controlling aversive reactions to chemotherapy, and lowering distress and enhancing well-being and quality of life (Jacobsen & Hann, 1998).

Cognitive–behavioral interventions teach individuals various active coping strategies (e.g., cognitive restructuring, relaxation, assertiveness) and are believed to enhance psychological functioning—especially in stressed individuals—by (a) modifying stressor appraisals and providing a coping response (Turk, Holzman, & Kerns, 1986), (b) changing maladaptive cognitive distortions (e.g., overgeneralizations, black-and-white thinking; A. D. Simons, Garfield, & Murphy, 1984), (c) decreasing hopeless thoughts (Rush, Beck, Kovacs, Weissenburger, & Hollon, 1982), and (d) increasing perceptions of self-efficacy, personal control, and mastery (Fishman & Loscalzo, 1987). As such, cognitive–behavioral interventions seem to be promising possibilities for addressing issues of personal control, coping, and hopelessness, which are key aspects of dealing with cancer.

Several studies have evaluated the use of cognitive–behavioral strategies with patients with cancer. Strategies include the use of progressive muscle relaxation (PMR) with patients who have colon cancer or melanoma (Levy, Herberman, & Whiteside, 1990); PMR, imagery, and biofeedback with patients who have metastatic cancers of mixed primary sites (Gruber et al., 1993); group-based multimodal CBSM for women with early- to mid-stage breast cancer (Andersen et al., 1998; Antoni et al., 2001); and structured, problem-oriented cognitive therapy (based on Beck's cognitive therapy for anxiety and depression) with patients with mixed cancer types (Greer et al., 1992). The latter program focuses on reducing anxiety and depressive symptoms and provides coping skills to help patients develop a "fighting spirit." The approach involves a cognitive model in which treatment goals are achieved by altering patients' appraisals about their disease and its accompanying events.

Other techniques often included under the rubric of cognitive–behavioral intervention for patients with cancer include contingency management, biofeedback, PMR, hypnosis, autogenic training, guided imagery, and stress inoculation training (Jacobsen & Hann, 1998). The majority of cognitive–behavioral interventions that have been tested empirically with patients with cancer have included combinations, or "packages," of these techniques, and many seem to include relaxation skills and tension reduction (e.g., progressive muscle, autogenics, guided imagery), coping-skills training, and problem-solving techniques (Jacobsen & Hann, 1998).

Some researchers have sought to explore the mechanisms by which these interventions facilitate adjustment. In one study, patients with stage I or II cancer who were participating in the 10-week, CBSM-based B-SMART intervention had a lower prevalence of moderate depression and experienced positive changes such as increased optimism and benefit finding (i.e., finding benefits in the cancer experience) as compared with control patients receiving a 1-day educational seminar. These positive changes remained significantly greater than those experienced by controls at least 9 months after the intervention (Antoni et al., 2001). Short-term increases in emotional processing (e.g., awareness, expression of emotions; Stanton, Kirk, Cameron, & Danoff-Burg, 2000) were observed during the first 10 weeks of the program and may be one of the ways that women make initial changes or breakthroughs. More specifically, not only did women in the B-SMART groups have increases in their awareness and expression of their feelings (compared with control women who did not change) but those who spent more time attempting to be aware and express their feelings during the 10 weeks of the intervention found more benefits in the cancer experience (Antoni et al., 2001). These intervention-associated improvements in adjustment may also have been facilitated by cognitive skills (e.g., cognitive restructuring and positive reframing) or social skills (e.g., assertive communications) taught during the intervention. Our prior work has indicated that changes in positive reframing and perceived social support may also explain many of the effects of CBSM-intervention-related improvements in mood, at least in patients with other medical conditions (Lutgendorf et al., 1998).

EXISTENTIAL/EXPERIENTIAL INTERVENTIONS

Another type of psychosocial intervention, often classified as *existential/experiential* group therapy and more recently as *supportive expressive therapy* (SET; Classen, Sandra, Sephton, Diamond, & Spiegel, 1998), also seems to have the potential to address the adjustment issues faced by people dealing with cancer. This intervention approach is designed to help individuals express and work through anxieties (e.g., death anxieties; Spiegel, & Glafkides, 1983) and express negative feelings, and it provides emotional support while encouraging individuals to pursue positive goals and activities. Some have suggested that these interventions offer the opportunity for group participants to share their strategies for dealing with cancer-related stressors, the chance for members to help one another, a sense of universality, and a buffer against the sense of isolation that many of them face (Spiegel et al., 1981; Yalom & Greaves, 1977). Thus, in theory, the existential/experiential interventions seem to address the issues of social isolation, emotional suppression, loss of self-esteem, and hopelessness that were mentioned previously. It is plausible, yet remains to be tested, that patients with early-stage disease (and a good prognosis) might benefit more from cognitive–behavioral intervention, whereas those with advanced metastatic disease might benefit more from SET group support programs that focus on pain management, existential challenges, and end-of-life issues (Fawzy & Fawzy, 1998).

Given that patients at different stages of disease may have issues that are more or less salient, it follows that certain types of intervention techniques may be more or less useful at different stages of the illness experience (Fawzy & Fawzy, 1998). For instance, when matching group-based therapy goals and methods to the stage of disease, a progression can be used as a guide: *prevention stage* (education intervention), *diagnosis stage* (education, coping-skills training, and emotional support interventions), *treatment stage* (coping, life adjustment, and emotional support interventions), *recovery stage* (active coping-skills training, emotional support, and reexamination of life goals interventions), *recurrence and dying stage* (active coping skills, pain and stress management, and existential therapy interventions), and *bereavement of family members* (emotional support and planning for the future interventions; Classen et al., 1998; Spira, 1997).

EMERGING INTERVENTION TARGETS

Fatigue and Sleep Problems

Many of the quality-of-life target areas in cancer highlighted in prior reviews involve anxiety symptoms and depressed mood (Payne, Hoffman, Theodoulou, Dosik, & Massie, 1999). Another area is persistent fatigue, clearly one of the most common experiences of patients treated for cancer (Portenoy & Miaskowski, 1998; Vogelzang et al., 1997). Cancer-related fatigue has many sources (Piper, Lindsey, & Dodd, 1991; Smets, Garssen, Schuster-Uitterhoeve, & de Haes, 1993; Winningham, Nail, & Burke, 1994), one of which is the medical and physical conditions associated with disease, surgery, and adjuvant treatment and concurrent systemic disorders (Portenoy & Miaskowski, 1998). Cancer-related fatigue may also stem from sleep disorders, lack of exercise, chronic pain, and use of centrally acting drugs (Engstrom, Strohl, Rose, Lewandowski, & Stefanek, 1999). Fatigue may also accompany anxiety or depressive states, and assessments capable of differentiating among these factors are important (Portenoy & Itri, 1999; Portenoy & Miaskowski, 1998). The factors just noted—anxiety, depression, fatigue, and sleep problems—likely exist in many patients with cancer and may be affected by psychosocial intervention. These phenomena may be influenced by focal concerns in the period after surgery such as fears about recurrence and potential damage from adjuvant therapy (Spencer et al., 1999). Interventions for helping people deal with these concerns may reduce fatigue and sleep disruptions by targeting mood management and reduction of tension and anxiety. Cognitive–behavioral techniques and relaxation training may be particularly effective strategies for dealing with these issues (Portenoy & Itri, 1999).

Surprisingly, almost no clinical trials have tested the efficacy of psychosocial interventions for decreasing or managing fatigue in patients with cancer. Pharmacological therapies may be warranted in patients with advanced disease and debilitating fatigue (Breitbart & Mermelstein, 1992; Bruera, Brenneis, Paterson, & MacDonald, 1989), but among patients with early- to mid-stage disease and moderate levels of fatigue who are returning to their home and work roles, nonpharmacological approaches may be equally effective. These approaches include patient education on the nature of symptoms and options for therapy (Winningham, 1996), supervised exercise and nutritional programs (MacVicar & Winningham,

1986), techniques that improve sleep hygiene and quality (Yellen & Dyonzak, 1996), and stress management and cognitive therapies (cf. Portenoy & Miaskowski, 1998).

A blend of education, tension and anxiety reduction, sleep monitoring, and cognitive restructuring may be an optimal package for reducing fatigue in patients with breast cancer in the period after surgery and during adjuvant therapy. These interventions may affect fatigue levels through a combination of stress management and improved sleep quality. It would be important to evaluate such an intervention package in controlled research designs because no study to date has tested the concurrent effects of such techniques on mood, fatigue, and sleep quality in patients with cancer during this period. If successful, this type of intervention could offer physical benefits. For instance, because research suggests that the influence of stressors and psychosocial factors on immune system functioning (e.g., NK cell counts, NKCC) may be mediated by alterations in sleep quality (Hall et al., 1998; Ironson et al., 1997; Irwin, Smith, & Gillin, 1992), it is still possible that psychosocial interventions for improving sleep quality may enhance health outcomes through psychoneuroimmunological mechanisms in people with cancer.

Pain

Another key quality-of-life issue for patients with cancer is pain and pain-related disruptions in daily functioning (Breitbart & Payne, 1998). Patients with early-stage breast cancer are not likely to have chronic pain or be receiving centrally acting opioid medications for pain in the weeks after surgery, but in patients with advanced disease, pain is likely to be a significant determinant of quality-of-life facets such as mood and sleep quality. Techniques such as hypnosis, relaxation and imagery, biofeedback, and music therapy have been found to be effective (Loscalzo & Jacobsen, 1990; Spiegel & Bloom, 1983).

Some of the key methodological issues that remain for studies evaluating the efficacy of psychosocial interventions for improving psychosocial adjustment in patients with cancer include (a) the need for a standardized, valid, and reliable set of assessment instruments to monitor changes and predictors of change in adjustment over time and (b) the need to use information on genetic factors (e.g., family cancer history), disease type and stage, treatment type and duration, demographic and sociocultural (e.g., ethnicity) factors, spiritual beliefs, and personality and contextual characteristics that could moderate intervention effects on adjustment. These sorts of research issues can only be addressed by large-scale clinical trials, and these trials are likely to be conducted in the next few years (Schneiderman, Antoni, Saab, & Ironson, 2001).

Optimizing Health Outcomes and Increasing Survival of Patients With Cancer

The targeted physical health benefits of psychosocial interventions in psycho-oncology can be grouped into at least three categories: (a) reducing cancer initiation and promotion, (b) preventing complications after treatment (e.g., immunosuppression, infectious disease, and other physical symptoms), and (c) lengthening disease-free survival time by slowing cancer progression.

REDUCING CANCER INITIATION AND PROMOTION

Because of the lack of evidence relating psychosocial factors to the development of cancer, no studies to date have studied the effects of psychosocial intervention on the initiation and promotion of cancers in high-risk hosts such as those who are immunocompromised (e.g., women with HIV infection, patients receiving immunosuppressive therapy after an organ transplant), those with a family history of cancer, or those who test positive for markers such as *BRCA* genes. Some target populations for future studies of interventions designed to reduce cancer promotion might include women testing positive for *BRCA* genes and women with stage 0 breast cancer (carcinoma in situ).

PREVENTING COMPLICATIONS AFTER TREATMENT

Stressors and surgery have been associated with decrements in immune functioning (van der Pompe, Antoni, & Heijnen, 1998), so stress-reducing psychosocial interventions administered just before breast cancer surgery might optimize the postsurgical immune status, possibly reducing the risk of infectious disease and possibly the growth of cancer cells that were mechanically spread through the surgical procedure. One recent pilot study showed that patients with breast cancer who receive two 90-minute sessions of information, problem-solving, relaxation exercises, and psychosocial support had a tendency to have lower declines in IFN-γ production by peripheral blood mononuclear cells after surgery than those receiving standard care (Larson, Duberstein, Talbot, Caldwell, & Moynihan, 2000). Although these results suggest that stress reduction techniques used before breast cancer surgery may help buffer the immune system during an otherwise potentially vulnerable period, the health implications of these findings are currently unclear.

One intriguing target for future psycho-oncology intervention research involves the proposed link between stress and susceptibility to infectious disease (Bovbjerg & Valdimarsdottir, 1996). It has been suggested that because stress is associated with increased susceptibility to upper respiratory infections (Cohen, Tyrrell, & Smith, 1991) and bacterial infections (Bovbjerg & Valdimarsdottir, 1996), patients with cancer, especially those who are emotionally distressed and receiving chemotherapy or other immunosuppressive adjuvant therapies, may be vulnerable to stress-associated opportunistic infections (Bovbjerg & Valdimarsdottir, 1996). These authors cite evidence that infectious disease is the leading cause of death in patients with cancer (White, 1993). Surprisingly, very little work has examined the effects of stressors or stress management interventions on the incidence of opportunistic infectious disease in patients receiving adjuvant therapy for cancer. This is likely to be an important area of exploration for psycho-oncology researchers in coming years. It is plausible that programs like B-SMART could be initiated some time after the breast cancer diagnosis and before patients undergo surgery. These studies are waiting to be done.

LENGTHENING DISEASE-FREE SURVIVAL TIME

The question of whether psychosocial interventions can affect the survival of patients with cancer and patients with other life-threatening diseases has been the subject of many reviews (e.g., Classen et al., 1998; Ironson, Antoni, & Lutgendorf, 1995). To date, at least seven studies using either random assignment or matched controls have tested the effects of psychosocial interventions on survival in patients with cancer (Classen et al., 1998). Among these studies, three seemed to improve survival time (Fawzy et al., 1993; Richardson et al., 1990; Spiegel et al., 1989), and four did not (Gellert, Maxwell, & Siegel, 1993; Goodwin et al., 2001; Ilnyckyj, Farber, Cheang, & Weinerman, 1994; M. Linn et al., 1982). In one of the set of studies, significant improvements in mood, phobic symptoms, maladaptive coping strategies, and pain were observed among patients with metastatic breast cancer participating in a 1-year SET group therapy intervention (Spiegel & Bloom, 1983). Moreover, after monitoring patients for 10 years, the investigators noted that the 50 women assigned to this intervention seemed to live, on average, twice as long as the 36 assigned to the standard of care condition (Spiegel et al., 1989). Richardson and colleagues found that among 94 patients with hematological malignancies, those assigned to any of three possible psychosocial conditions (each involving education about treatment side effects and the importance of compliance and self-care) had a greater survival time at 2- to 5-year follow-ups (Richardson et al., 1990). Finally, one study showed that among 68 patients diagnosed with early-stage malignant melanoma, those assigned to a 6-week structured stress management group had a significantly longer survival time and a marginally significantly longer time to recurrence during the 5- to 6-year follow-up than those receiving standard care (Fawzy et al., 1993). Two of the studies revealing no survival effects were randomized trials using patients with cancers of different sites and stages (Ilnyckyj et al., 1994; M. Linn et al., 1982), whereas the third study used patients with breast cancer and matched control patients (Gellert et al., 1993). The fourth study, which was the most recently published, examined the effects of group-based SET in a randomized trial of 235 women with metastatic breast cancer (Goodwin et al., 2001). Although the SET intervention was successful in decreasing mood disturbance and pain reports, it had no effect on survival in the 6-year follow-up period.

DISCREPANCIES IN CANCER SURVIVAL STUDIES

Considering their discrepancies, what firm conclusions can be drawn from the cancer survival studies? Before answering this question, it is prudent to align the studies according to methodological grounds. The seven studies involved interventions with different theoretical orientations, different lengths, and different formats (group vs. individual); involved follow-up periods ranging from 1 to 11 years; and included patients dealing with a wide variety of cancer types at varying stages of disease. These methodological differences make it very difficult to compare results across studies.

If one focuses on the two studies that are the most alike—the Goodwin et al. (2001) study and the Spiegel et al. (1989) study—some similarities are apparent. Both studies used group-based SET intervention for women with metastatic breast cancer, and both studies reported significant effects of the intervention on psychological status and pain reports. However, although the Spiegel et al. study found significant effects of the intervention on survival time, the Goodwin et al. study did not. Aside from the Goodwin study having a shorter follow-up period than Spiegel's (6 vs. 10 years), the differences between the studies are not readily apparent. However, it is possible that the slight differences in age and menopausal status between the intervention and control groups could have obscured some differences in the Goodwin et al. study, although this is unlikely because the results were the same when these extraneous factors were controlled.

Another possibility is that treatment improvements available during the Goodwin study period (1993 to 1998) not in place during the time of the Spiegel study (early 1980s) may have made it more difficult to detect a difference in survival. This limitation could have been compounded by the shorter follow-up period used in the Goodwin et al. study. It is interesting that in two other studies of psychosocial interventions for patients with metastatic breast cancer conducted during this time, a similar lack of effect on survival was noted (Cunningham et al., 1998; S. Edelman, Bell, & Kidman, 1999). Note that these studies used much smaller samples and nonrandomized designs.

In addition, among women assigned to the control condition in the Goodwin et al. (2001) study, more than 10% sought out support groups outside of the study protocol. Although slightly greater than the number in the intervention group who sought such outside support, this difference was not significant but does suggest a 1990s trend that may not have been relevant in the early 1980s when Spiegel conducted his trial. It may suggest that the general population was more aware of the need for psychological support among patients dealing with advanced breast cancer. In this book, we have emphasized that even women with less advanced breast cancer can significantly benefit from a psychosocial intervention. We are currently in the process of studying the longer term psychological and physical health effects of the B-SMART intervention among women who are at an early stage of disease when they receive the intervention to address this issue.

Classen et al. (1998) have suggested that common factors may exist among the interventions producing significant effects on survival but are relatively absent in the studies failing to duplicate this finding. They identified these factors as (a) the inclusion of patients with the same type and stage of cancer within each group (which fosters commonality, normalizes the disease experience, and addresses shared concerns), (b) the creation of a supportive environment (which provides social support and the opportunity for emotional expression), (c) the inclusion of an educational component (which decreases uncertainty and increases feelings of control), and (d) the provision of stress management and coping skills training (which decreases arousal and distress, models coping strategies, increases self-efficacy). All of these features were incorporated into the development and evaluation of our B-SMART program. Currently, several research programs in the United States and abroad are investigating the effects of psychosocial interventions on quality of life and survival time in patients with breast cancer (Classen et al., 1998). It seems worthwhile that these investigators are attempting to control for factors such as sample homogeneity and are including supportive, educational, and skill-building elements in their intervention protocols. These steps will facilitate comparisons of efficacy and effect sizes across the many centers participating in this line of research in coming years.

Biobehavioral Mechanisms for Health Effects of Psychosocial Interventions

Some have proposed that the factors mediating the health effects of these interventions may be grouped into three broad categories: (a) negative health behaviors (e.g., smoking, increased fat intake), (b) enhancement of positive health behaviors (e.g., diet, exercise, medical adherence), and (c) modulation of biological systems (e.g., neuroendocrine and immune systems; Baum & Posluszny, 1999; Classen et al., 1998). However, very little research has evaluated any of these as mediators of the interventions that have been shown to affect survival in patients with cancer.

Andersen et al. (1994) formulated a biobehavioral model with psychological, behavioral, and biological paths relating stress to cancer disease course. They argued that cancer diagnosis and treatment may induce acute and chronic stress and reduce quality of life. These changes may be accompanied or followed by poor compliance to medical regimens, increases in negative health behaviors, decreases in positive health behaviors, and irregular neuroendocrine and immune functioning, possibly contributing to local and metastatic disease progression. As Andersen et al. (1994) noted, research at the interface of behavioral oncology and immunology has methodological challenges. They recommended that studies use an experimental design, focus on a specific cancer type and stage (favoring certain types—breast, ovary and cervix, and prostate—and early stages rather than later stages), and use participants who have homogeneous, well-established clinicopathological prognostic factors (e.g., nodal status, estrogen and progesterone receptor status, and menopausal status for patients with breast cancer; Clark & McGuire, 1992; van der Pompe et al., 1994).

Very few studies have examined the relationship between immune system changes and stressors specifically experienced by patients with breast cancer. Among patients with stage I or II breast cancer, Levy et al. (1987) found that elevated distress after surgery predicted lower NKCC 15 months after surgery, and lower NKCC at this time predicted a shorter time to recurrence in the 5- to 8-year follow-up. Among these patients, greater NKCC was also related to patients' perceptions of greater emotional support from their spouse, greater perceived support from their physician, and seeking social support as a coping strategy (Levy et al., 1990). Levy et al. (1991) also found that elevated distress predicted less time to recurrence among those patients with stage I or II breast cancer who had disease progression after treatment. It might be hypothesized that distress, poor coping strategies, and perceptions of low social sup-

Impact of Psychological Factors on Health: More Research Needed

More data are needed on the physiological impact of psychological changes during diagnosis and treatment for cancer and the physiological impact of a psychosocial intervention during this period. Newly treated patients with cancer are vulnerable to distress and a decrease in the number of their positive experiences (van der Pompe et al., 1994), possibly decreasing cellular immune functions (Herbert & Cohen, 1993a, 1993b) that survey the development of metastases (Andersen, Farrar, et al., 1998; Andersen, Kiecolt-Glaser, & Glaser, 1994). Thus, psychosocial interventions may provide mental and physical health benefits, with the physical benefits potentially being mediated by intervention-associated changes in specific endocrine and immune functions (Andersen et al., 1994; Ironson et al., 1995). Psychosocial interventions may also facilitate positive adaptations (e.g., enhanced relationships, positive emotional growth) that have direct effects on immune system functions such as NKCC (Levy et al., 1990).

port during the period after surgery could contribute to persisting decrements in immune function, thereby possibly increasing the risk of regional and distant micrometastases over longer periods.

One strategy for examining such associations might be to study changes in positive experiences (e.g., finding benefits in the cancer experience, having an increased sense of meaning, developing spirituality), distress, physical quality of life, social support, cognitive and behavioral coping strategies, and immune status in patients with cancer during the course of a psychosocial intervention designed to change these psychosocial variables. We have reasoned that it would be best to conduct this study during a stressful point in patients' treatment, shortly after surgery, or after adjuvant therapy has been completed and monitor participants over time for psychosocial, immune, and health changes. It is arguable that any stress- or intervention-associated changes in immune status during this period may have the greatest health implications for patients with lower basal immune functioning from surgery, chemotherapy, and radiation.

BENEFICIAL IMPACT OF PSYCHOSOCIAL INTERVENTIONS ON THE IMMUNE SYSTEM

Relaxation and guided imagery have been shown to modulate lymphocyte proliferative response to challenge and NKCC in healthy patients

(Kiecolt-Glaser et al., 1986; Kiecolt-Glaser, Glaser, & Williger, 1985; Zachariae, Hansen, & Andersen, 1994). Kiecolt-Glaser et al. (1985) found a 30% increase in NKCC after 1 month of muscle relaxation training among healthy adults living in a retirement home. Combining cognitive stress management with relaxation training can enhance psychological well-being and modulate immune functioning in people dealing with a new medical diagnosis or its treatment (Antoni et al., 1991; Esterling et al., 1992; Fawzy et al., 1993). Fawzy et al. (1993) showed that after surgery, patients with malignant melanoma who received a 6-week group psychosocial intervention used more of the active coping strategies (Fawzy, Cousins, et al., 1990) and had higher interferon-stimulated NKCC than those who had surgery and standard care only (Fawzy, Kemeny, et al., 1990). Interestingly, the more the patients increased active coping during the intervention, the greater their likelihood of surviving at the 6-year follow-up (Fawzy et al., 1993).

Studies examining similar phenomena in patients with breast cancer have been based on smaller samples but obtained evidence that time-limited stress management interventions can modulate immune system indexes in women with early-stage breast cancer. Schedlowski, Jungk, Schimanski, Tewes, and Schmoll (1994) found decreases in plasma cortisol and increases in numbers of circulating lymphocytes in patients with early-stage breast cancer who completed a 10-week intervention consisting of relaxation and guided imagery. Gruber et al. (1993) found that 13 patients with early-stage breast cancer who completed a 9-week stress reduction intervention had increases in lymphocyte proliferative responses and NKCC. One report of an ongoing psychosocial intervention study of patients with breast cancer noted significant distress reductions and better quality of life accompanied by increases in NKCC among 100 patients with stage II or III disease who participated in an intervention group designed to reduce stress, enhance quality of life, and increase positive health behaviors and decrease negative ones (Andersen, 1998; Andersen, Golden-Kreutz, & Farrar, 1997). One study of 23 patients with breast cancer who had positive axillary nodes or distant metastases found that those in a 13-week group-based psychosocial intervention had significant increases in lymphocyte proliferative responses to challenge (14%) compared with a wait-list group, which had 33% decrements in the same period (van der Pompe, Duivenvoorden, Antoni, Visser, & Heijnen, 1997).

In the most recent report in this series, our group found that patients with breast cancer assigned to the 10-week B-SMART program had significant increases in lymphocyte proliferative responses to anti-CD3 stimulation (McGregor et al., 2000). Note that women who were able to find more benefits in the cancer experience (including an increased sense of the meaning of life, improved interpersonal relationships, and greater spirituality) during the 10-week intervention period had greater lymphocyte proliferative responses 3 months after the conclusion of the intervention. This is relevant in that increases in benefit finding were found to mediate the effects of this intervention in decreasing cortisol levels during the 10-week treatment period (Cruess, Antoni, McGretor et al., 2000). Although recent work has related positive affect states to decreased cortisol levels (Buchanan, al'Absi, & Lovallo, 1999), this is the first work to show that increases in perceived positive gains may explain some of the effects of a psychosocial intervention such as B-SMART on cortisol reductions and increases in lymphocyte proliferation in women with breast cancer. Thus, preliminary studies support the hypothesis that time-limited psychosocial interventions may modulate immune system functioning in people with breast cancer. Many of the immune measures shown to change during these interventions may be relevant to the course of certain cancers, though no work to date has linked these immunological changes to disease outcomes in patients with cancer.

Moreover, all of the psychosocial intervention research of patients with cancer has focused on unspecific indexes of immune system status, which make it difficult to draw conclusions about prospective mechanisms of immune system regulation (e.g., determining how cell-signaling cytokines such as IFN-γ change and how these changes relate to psychosocial changes during intervention). Furthermore, the health relevance of intervention-related immune changes remains unknown, so long-term follow-up studies of the women who have participated in these trials are needed. This work is ongoing.

In summary, with the exception of the work of Fawzy et al. (1993), no study to date has examined the underlying psychoneuroimmunology mechanisms that may account for the effect of psychosocial factors on health outcomes (disease recurrence and mortality) in patients dealing with cancer. It is plausible that stress hormones released through SNS and HPAC activation, which occur during distress states and down-regulate immune system functioning, are potential sources of physiological mediators that may help elucidate the connection between psychological processes and disease progression. Some patients with cancer have had elevated levels of cortisol (Grinevich & Labunetz, 1986), which may be caused by disease-related processes or may be a by-product of distress states after surgery and initial treatment. It may be that distress states and stress hormone levels change simultaneously during the initial stages of disease before the habituation of HPAC axis functioning common in people with chronic or advanced disease states. In any event, these alterations in stress hormones may also have a direct impact on the immune system's ability to battle infection, which may then subsequently affect long-term health outcomes and disease course in people dealing with cancer and its challenging treatments.

Future studies need to explore neuroendocrine mediators of psycho-social, health, and immune status among patients with different types of cancer. For certain hormonally mediated cancers such as breast cancer, it is important to explore the possibility that intervention effects on health outcomes are mediated by sex hormones (e.g., testosterone and estro-gens) as well as the classic adrenal stress hormones such as cortisol. The B-SMART intervention was recently shown to decrease testosterone lev-els in women with early-stage breast cancer (D. Cruess, Antoni, McGregor, et al., 2000). Given that higher testosterone levels are associated with greater risk for breast cancer, this decrease may signify the ability of the intervention to normalize HPG levels.

THE FUTURE OF PSYCHOSOCIAL INTERVENTION RESEARCH OF PATIENTS WITH BREAST CANCER

Psychosocial interventions have been shown to modulate NKCC (Andersen et al., 1997), lymphocyte proliferative responses to challenge (van der Pompe, Duivenvoorden, et al., 1997), and lymphocyte number (Schedlowski et al., 1994) and reduce circulating cortisol levels (Cruess, Antoni, McGregor, et al., 2000; Schedlowski et al., 1994; van der Pompe, Duivenvoorden, et al., 1997) in varying stages of breast cancer. A widely publicized study also demonstrated that patients with metastatic breast cancer assigned to a long-term SET group intervention lived twice as long as similar women assigned to standard care (Spiegel et al, 1989). It is possible that the opportunity for emotional expression, processing and assimilation, and social support offered during this intervention contrib-uted to the greater longevity. However, no immunological or endocrine measurements were collected during this study, thus psychoneuroimmunological mechanisms can only be theorized to ex-plain these effects. Moreover, efforts to replicate the health effects of SET intervention in patients with metastatic breast cancer have not yet been successful (e.g., Goodwin et al., 2001).

Although more and more studies are able to demonstrate psycho-neuroimmunological associations with stress and distress in patients with different types of cancer, the health relevance of these associations is still largely unknown. It has been suggested that according to these studies, psychosocial factors are more likely to be associated with disease course in younger women and those with the early stages of disease (Schultz, Bookwala, Knapp, Scheier, &Williamson, 1996). It is known that younger women are more likely than older women to have more aggressive breast cancer or to be diagnosed with a higher grade of breast cancer and to have extensive axillary lymph node metastases (Pratap & Shousha, 1998), suggesting that the possible health benefits from successful intervention may be greater in younger women. It is widely accepted that psycho-neuroimmunological research of patients with cancer needs to control for factors such as age, type and stage of disease, and ongoing adjuvant therapies such as chemotherapy, radiation, hormonal therapy, and immunotherapy because each of them can have a significant effect on immunological measures such as NKCC (Tichatschek et al., 1988). Studies that do so may help clarify this aspect of research.

On the basis of the research just summarized, immune system factors such as NKCC, lymphocyte proliferative responses to challenge, and lymphocyte subpopulations involved with helper T-cell function and cytotoxic T-cell function may play a role in (a) the initiation or promotion of neoplastic disease processes in patients who are at risk because of a decrease in immunosuppression or in those who a genetically predisposed for disease. These immune factors may also influence (b) the recurrence of disease in patients who have undergone curative and adjuvant treatments (e.g., women with breast cancer) through their putative ability to monitor cancer cells that have spread to areas beyond the primary organ site (e.g., breast) to another type of tissue (e.g., bone, lung, brain). Important elements of a comprehensive immune battery for this line of work to evaluate the effects of the interventions being used for patients with breast cancer would include measures of lymphocyte proliferation and phenotypes for CD4+ T helper cells, CD8+ cytotoxic T cells, NK cells, dendritic cells, macrophages, and B cells and cytokine-stimulated NKCC toward standard targets and specific breast cancer cell lines. One strategy for examining such associations is to study changes in quality of life and physical health of patients with cancer during the course of an intervention designed to change psychosocial variables such as social support and cognitive and behavioral coping strategies. These intervention-associated changes may be accompanied by changes in HPAC and SNS hormonal activity and immune system functions such as NKCC, which may have implications for the physical health and survival of these various patient groups. It is plausible that any stress-induced changes in immune status during this period may have the greatest health implications for patients with lower basal immune functioning because of recent surgery or adjuvant therapy.

Conclusion

In summary, during the past 20 years, psycho-oncological research has increased at a dramatic pace, involving a proliferation of different research designs and an attempt to generalize findings to several types of cancer. However, with this quantitative growth has come a large collection of inconsistent findings. These inconsistencies may be attributed partly to (a) differences in the nature of the psychosocial independent variables used (e.g., psychosocial predictors and interventions) and a lack of theory-driven models to guide hypothesis formulation, (b) heterogeneity of the cancers chosen for study, and (c) inconsistencies in intervention-associated psychosocial and biomedical outcome measures evaluated. The possible mechanisms underlying the relationships between behavior and cancer are undoubtedly complex. Without a theory-driven model to guide the construction of interventions for modulating these relationships, any findings ascertained are difficult to interpret and very hard to replicate. Our theoretical model of how the B-SMART intervention may affect quality of life and physical health inpatients with breast cancer is explained in the next chapter.

Psycho-oncological models that describe the power of psychosocial characteristics and psychosocial intervention to predict cancer outcomes can greatly reduce the number of variables studied and thus improve the efficiency of the scientific research process and the likely effectiveness of clinical intervention efforts. Theory-driven models give rise to classification rules for logically related variables (e.g., coping strategies, which are categorized as active or passive and emotion or problem focused). This helps researchers select variables, clarify testable hypotheses, place real limits on the phenomena (e.g., tumor type and stage) likely to go through the course of events prescribed by the model, and dictate the design features necessary to test the relationships predicted (e.g., timing and number of assessments required to capture meaningful changes during an intervention).

Research has shown that psychological stress can contribute to decreased immune system functioning in different forms of cancers, including breast cancer (Andersen et al., 1998). Other research has demonstrated that cognition (e.g., attitudes, appraisals, values), coping strategies, and social support can influence psychological distress states and contribute to positive health outcomes in patients with breast cancer (Watson et al., 1999). Finally, psychosocial interventions such as CBSM have been shown to affect mood states (positive and negative) and quality of life (Trijsburg et al., 1992); SNS (e.g., norepinephrine), adrenocortical (e.g., cortisol), and adrenal gonadal (testosterone, dehydroepiandrosterone-S [DHEA-S]) neuroendocrine hormones; and immune system functioning in patients with different diseases including breast cancer (Cruess, Antoni, McGregor, et al., 2000, Cruess, Antoni, McGregor, et al., 2001; McGregor et al., 2000) and HIV infection (Antoni, Cruess, Wagner, et al., 2000; Antoni, Wagner, et al., 2000; Cruess et al., 1999; Cruess, Antoni, Schneiderman, et al., 2000; Lutgendorf et al., 1997). Furthermore, our work has shown that these types of interventions may induce these psychological and physiological changes by increasing relaxation and altering tension and anxiety levels, cognitions (e.g., appraisals, benefit finding, optimism), coping strategies (e.g., acceptance, positive reframing), and social support (S. Cruess, Antoni, Cruess, et al., 2000; D. Cruess, Antoni, McGregor, et al., 2000; Lutgendorf et al., 1998; McGregor et al., 2000).

Future psycho-oncology research involved in behavioral management of patients with cancer should build on and expand the scientific foundation and ultimately evaluate the efficacy and effectiveness of psychosocial interventions designed to improve mood, quality of life, and physical health of patients who are dealing with different types of cancer. Chapter 2 describes the 10 years of empirical research that was integral in developing and validating the psychosocial intervention we designed for women dealing with breast cancer.

Empirical Research With the B-SMART Program | 2

A series of systematic research projects were undertaken during the past 10 years to develop and evaluate the intervention that we developed: the *Breast Cancer Stress Management And Relaxation Training*, or B-SMART, program. In this chapter, I summarize the results of studies that (a) identified the major concerns of women with early-stage breast cancer, which helped us tailor aspects of the intervention to the needs of women with breast cancer; (b) documented key psychosocial variables involved in vulnerability and resilience, or "mediators" of adjustment (i.e., personality and contextual variables involved in the effects of vulnerability and resilience factors on emotional and social well-being after surgery); and (c) identified medical and demographic factors indicating which patients are likely to pursue complementary and alternative therapies and psychosocial services after a diagnosis of breast cancer. All of these studies were useful in identifying the key elements that we needed to include in the B-SMART program.

I also present a final set of studies comprising randomized clinical trials designed to test the efficacy of the B-SMART program for modifying emotional adjustment and indicators of physiological regulation (endocrine and immune function) in women with early-stage breast cancer. Each research area involves a key question we hoped to address. The following descriptions of each study are preceded with the key questions and a bulleted list of the research articles that we believe best answer the questions.

What Are the Chief Concerns of Women With Early-Stage Breast Cancer?

▍ "Concerns of a Multi-Ethnic Sample of Early Stage Breast Cancer Patients and Relations to Psychosocial Well-Being" (Spencer et al., 1999).

To best tailor our intervention program to meet the needs of women with breast cancer, we conducted a study designed to identify the major concerns that women have during the months after surgery, a time when many of them are undergoing adjuvant treatments such as chemotherapy and radiation. The primary aim of this study was to determine which concerns were most salient to patients with breast cancer—to fine-tune the content of the B-SMART program. Therefore, we developed the Profile of Concerns About Breast Cancer (PCBC). The PCBC (see display) surveys a wide variety of concerns in several domains, ranging from existential issues such as recurrence, pain, and premature death to practical issues such as bills, social issues such as adverse reactions from family and friends, work issues such as discrimination in hiring, and sexual issues such as the loss of a sense of femininity and sexual feelings.

The PCBC was completed by 223 patients with early-stage breast cancer (48 Hispanic, 24 African American, 151 Caucasian) within 1 year of their diagnosis and treatment. The profile reported by younger women differed from that of older women, primarily in that their level of concern was higher overall. For the most part, the concerns that were rated as "high" (i.e., most important) were consistent among all ages. The issue that concerned women the most was *recurrence* (3.14 among all women on a 1 to 5 scale, 3.39 among younger women). After recurrence, concerns involved being sick or damaged by adjuvant therapy, not seeing their children grow, premature death, and life with their partner being cut short. Issues of moderate concern involved loss of sexual desirability and sexual feelings. The issues of least intense concern involved adverse reactions from others. The various concerns aggregated into three broad areas: (a) life and pain, (b) sexuality, and (c) rejection. Multiple regression analyses revealed that life and pain issues and sexuality issues were unique in the way that they predicted emotional distress, sexual disruption, and impairment in the women's sense of femininity. Life and pain issues and rejection issues were unique in the way that they predicted social disruption.

We also found ethnic differences in the concerns reported and adverse reactions expressed. Hispanic women reported more intense con-

Items From the PCBC

As you think about your illness, how much are you concerned . . .

1. that you won't be able to get a better job (or be promoted) if they know you had cancer?
2. that you won't be given the raises you deserve because of your illness?
3. that the bills from the treatment will be overwhelming?
4. that you won't be able to have children?
5. that you won't see your children grow up?
6. that your partner (or a potential new partner) will reject you because of the cancer or your treatment?
7. that your children will become less affectionate or less loving with you?
8. that your family will become angry with you?
9. that you will argue more with your partner?
10. that the treatment will make you feel less feminine, less like a woman?
11. that the treatment will make you less desirable sexually?
12. that the various treatments will make you less likely to have sexual feelings?
13. that people won't think you look as good as you did?
14. that your friends will avoid you?
15. that people at work won't want to interact with you?
16. that your friends will act as though your disease is contagious?
17. that chemotherapy or radiation therapy will make you sick?
18. that chemotherapy or radiation therapy will damage your body in some way?
19. that you'll undergo an early menopause?
20. that you may die soon?
21. that you won't be able to go places you want to go and do things you want to do?
22. that you will always feel physically damaged from this disease?
23. that your life with your partner will be cut short?
24. that the cancer may come back?
25. that you will lose your sense of independence and self-sufficiency?
26. that others perceive you as less strong, fit, and healthy than before you were diagnosed with breast cancer?

(Continued)

27. that physical pain might come from your illness or its treatment?
28. that you might become dependent on or addicted to drugs or medications?
29. that your daughter or granddaughter may develop breast cancer too?

cerns of various types than did other women, as well as higher levels of emotional distress and social and sexual disruption. African American women reported lower levels of distress and disruption of their sense of femininity than did the other groups.

We also found relationships between the three areas of concerns and vulnerability factors such as optimism, social support, and body image. Women with more concerns in the life and pain area and sexuality area were less optimistic, had less social support, and were more invested in body integrity as a source of self-acceptance. Less social support and a greater investment in body integrity were also related to rejection issues. Investment in appearance related to more concerns about sexuality issues.

These findings helped us define numerous areas of focus for intervention. Cognitive coping responses and positive thinking (optimism) constitute one such focus. We also found that we needed to help women develop relaxation skills to help them deal with pain, cope with the side effects of adjuvant treatment, and avoid medication dependence. The third area is the need to focus on maintenance and enhancement of social contacts, which involves assertiveness training to help women explain to their family and friends ways they are being helpful and ways they are not. Finally, we found that the intervention should itself serve as a source of emotional support. A supportive group should help its members resist the urge to withdraw from other sources of support and other aspects of their normal, everyday life.

Which Psychosocial Factors Influence the Adjustment Process?

- ▪ "Effects of Mastectomy vs. Lumpectomy on Emotional Adjustment to Breast Cancer" (Pozo et al., 1992).
- ▪ "Optimism vs. Pessimism Predicts the Quality of Women's Adjustment to Early Stage Breast Cancer" (Carver et al., 1994).

- "How Important Is the Perception of Personal Control? Studies of Early Stage Breast Cancer Patients" (Carver, Harris, et al., 2000).
- "Responsiveness to Threats and Incentives, Expectations of Cancer Recurrence, and the Experiences of Emotional Distress and Disengagement: Moderator Effects in a Sample of Early-Stage Breast Cancer Patients" (Carver, Meyer, & Antoni, 2000).
- "Distress and Internalized Homophobia Among Lesbian Women Treated for Early-Stage Breast Cancer" (McGregor, Antoni, Alferi, & Carver, 2001).

A woman's adjustment after surgery for breast cancer may be predicted by her choice of surgical technique (i.e., mastectomy vs. lumpectomy; Pozo et al., 1992). Women receiving a lumpectomy may have less distress during and after the surgery. However, it is now known that personality and social context predispose some people to be more responsive to problems inherent in the diagnosis and treatment of breast cancer—and these factors are independent of the surgery experiences themselves. These factors can be thought of as vulnerability and resilience factors and include optimism, expectations of disease recurrence, sensitivity to potential threats and rewards resulting from the decision-making process, and investment in body image.

OPTIMISM

One vulnerability/resilience variable we examined was optimism. Much evidence shows that optimists and pessimists handle adversity with differing levels of success (Scheier & Carver, 1992). This work assessed optimism as expectancies for good versus bad outcomes in one's life. Optimists respond to difficulties by exerting effort, whereas pessimists tend to give up. The act of giving up is accompanied by greater distress in pessimists (Carver & Scheier, 1990), and this effect has been noted by numerous researchers (for review, see Scheier & Carver, 1992). Optimism confers similar benefits for women who have been diagnosed with or are undergoing surgery for breast cancer (Carver et al., 1993, 1994). Optimism (which was assessed before surgery) indicated that a woman would have less emotional distress during the first year after surgery. Optimism also predicted resistance to the development of distress during the months after surgery. That is, controlling for the prior association between pessimism and distress, pessimism predicted higher later distress.

EXPECTATION OF CANCER RECURRENCE

- "How Important Is the Perception of Personal Control? Studies of Early Stage Breast Cancer Patients" (Carver, Harris, et al., 2000).

■ "Responsiveness to Threats and Incentives, Expectations of Cancer Recurrence, and the Experiences of Emotional Distress and Disengagement: Moderator Effects in a Sample of Early-Stage Breast Cancer Patients" (Carver, Meyer, & Antoni, 2000).

Theory and research hold that expectancies relate to emotional and behavioral responses to adversity (e.g., Bandura, 1986; Carver et al., 1993; Carver & Scheier, 1998; Litt, Tennen, Affleck, & Klock, 1992; Scheier & Carver, 1992). People with confidence about the future respond to adverse experiences (whether chronic illness, a diagnosis of a life-threatening disease, or a natural disaster) by trying to move forward with their lives, and they have low levels of emotional distress compared with people who are not confident about the future. People who are doubtful about the future tend to give up when they confront adversity. They also become more distressed as long as goal commitment remains. We have shown that expecting to remain cancer free in the future predicts better emotional adjustment among newly treated patients with breast cancer (Carver, Harris, et al., 2000).

The detrimental effects of doubt about the future may be magnified for someone who is very responsive to threats but minor for a person who is not very threat sensitive. Similarly, the detrimental effects of doubt may be especially pronounced among people who are not motivated by a sensitive reward (incentive-pursuit) system but less important among those who respond more strongly to incentives. The diagnosis of breast cancer is a threatening and an unsettling event (Derogatis, 1986; S. E. Taylor, 1983) because patients face the prospect of dying or becoming permanently disfigured. A host of difficult existential and pragmatic questions and concerns inevitably surface (Spencer et al., 1999) in the patient's mind: "Has (or will) the cancer spread? Will my sense of femininity be irreparably damaged? Will friends and family react poorly? How will adjuvant therapy affect me? What sort of financial impact will the treatment have on me?"

We examined distress and giving up among 220 women who had been treated for breast cancer within the past year. We hypothesized that these women would exhibit more distress and behavioral disengagement—a giving-up response—if they were threat sensitive. Furthermore, we hypothesized that their reactions to threats would be magnified by doubts about whether they would remain cancer free in the future, which is the single greatest concern of these patients (Spencer et al., 1999). Indeed, we found that those who were threat sensitive by nature and believed the cancer would return would report disproportionately high distress and disengagement (Carver, Meyer, & Antoni, 2000). Therefore, personality characteristics that cause women to focus on threats in their lives may make them particularly prone to adjustment difficulties after a diagnosis of cancer—a situation that may be amplified among women who perceive that they are or who have been told that they are at high risk for recurrence. For these women, cognitive–behavioral (CBSM) techniques that challenge the cognitive appraisals underlying threatening circumstances surrounding the cancer experience (rational thought replacement) may help to circumvent these tendencies.

INVESTMENT IN BODY IMAGE

Another vulnerability factor we have studied is the dependence of self-esteem on body image. We hypothesized that women whose self-acceptance depends heavily on body image would be especially vulnerable to psychosocial disruption after surgery for breast cancer (Carver et al., 1998). (We studied two aspects of body image: (a) self-acceptance dependent on appearance and (b) self-acceptance dependent on a sense of body integrity and wholeness. We reasoned that a diagnosis of breast cancer challenges a person's self-image. Surgery creates a disruptive physical change and disruptive change in the sense of physical health and implicit feelings of invulnerability. We found that women who reported a strong investment in the integrity of their bodies reported disrupted social interaction at follow-ups and a stronger sense of alienation from themselves (i.e., "not feeling like myself anymore"). Women who reported a strong investment in looking good experienced more emotional distress.

SEXUAL IDENTITY

For women who identify themselves as lesbians, aspects of their attitudes toward homosexuality may affect their emotional adjustment after surgery (McGregor et al., 2000). Because having positive feelings about oneself as a homosexual has been related to better mental health in male homosexuals (Meyer & Dean, 1995), we hypothesized that positive feelings about oneself as a homosexual (i.e., lower internalized homophobia) would relate to better mental health among lesbians. Because internalized homophobia has been linked to lower self-esteem and social support among gay men (Nicholson & Long, 1990; Ross & Rosser, 1996), we used path analysis to examine whether self-esteem and perceived social support could mediate between internalized homophobia and emotional well-being. A convenience sample of 57 lesbians who had been recruited for a study of adjustment to breast cancer completed measures of internalized homophobia, degree of disclosure of sexual orientation, social support, self-esteem, and distress. In keeping with predictions, internalized homophobia related to greater distress. Path models were consistent with the theory that internalized homophobia promotes distress through lower self-esteem and lower perceived social support. However, the data were also consistent with a model in which low self-esteem leads to internalized homophobia by way of elevated distress. Internalized homophobia also related inversely to use of health care resources. Similar to our findings for investment in body image, the ways that women conceptualize themselves sexually or physically may contribute in important ways to their ability to adjust emotionally to breast cancer diagnosis and treatment.

This pattern of results, combined with the results of our studies on optimism and pessimism and expectancies about cancer recurrence, suggests that cognitive factors may play a very large role in determining how well women adjust during the breast cancer experience. It also suggests that interventions addressing cognitive appraisals (e.g., CBSM) may be important in facilitating the adjustment process for these women.

Mediating Factors: Which Underlying Psychological Mechanisms Explain the Link Between Resilience/ Vulnerability Factors and Adjustment?

- ▪ "How Coping Mediates the Effects of Optimism on Distress: A Study of Women With Early Stage Breast Cancer" (Carver et al., 1993).
- ▪ "Religiosity, Religious Coping, and Distress: A Prospective Study of Catholic and Evangelical Hispanic Women in Treatment for Early Stage Breast Cancer" (Alferi, Culver, Carver, Arena, & Antoni, 1999).
- ▪ "An Exploratory Study of Social Support, Distress, and Disruption Among Low Income Hispanic Women Under Treatment for Early Stage Breast Cancer" (Alferi, Carver, Antoni, Weiss, & Duran, 2001).

The coping responses of women with breast cancer play an important role in how successfully they adjust to having the disease (Carver et al., 1993) and may explain the reason optimists generally fare better than pessimists. During the period just before and the months after surgery, we studied a group of women with early-stage breast cancer. Women completed the COPE, an index of 13 different coping strategies used to deal with the breast cancer experience (Carver, Scheier, & Weintraub, 1989), and a distress measure at each time point in this study. Although dysfunctional coping was not frequent, it was important. Greater distress experiences related to denial and disengagement at numerous points (see

TABLE 2.1

Correlations of Coping Responses With Distress

Coping response	Before surgery	After surgery	3-month follow-up	6-month follow-up	12-month follow-up
Denial	.70	.66	.46	.39	.42
Behavioral disengagement	.55	.53	.40	.37	.30
Acceptance	−.68	−.47	−.29	−.43	−.27
Positive reframing	−.48	−.26	−.27	−.30	[−.14]
Use of humor	[−.20]	−.34	[−.20]	−.41	[−.13]
Use of religion	[.04]	[−.04]	[.00]	[.06]	[.03]

Note. Bracketed values do not attain significance by two-tailed test.

Table 2.1). Denial and disengagement coping also prospectively predicted the development of distress over time.

Other aspects of coping had more favorable implications (see Table 2.1). Of greatest interest is the effect of accepting the situation's reality. Acceptance related to better adaptation at all points. Also associated with better adjustment were positive reframing and humor. Acceptance was also a significant prospective predictor of less distress (controlling for prior distress levels) during the period after surgery.

The data also indicated that coping responses are a mediator through which optimism influences adjustment. Not surprisingly, optimists and pessimists coped differently. Optimists accepted the fact that the situation had to be handled, positively reframed the situation, and moved forward. Pessimists tried to push the experience away and when unable to do so tended to give up goals threatened by the diagnosis and surgery. Results of path analyses suggested that differences in coping explained a large part of the effects of optimism on distress (Carver et al., 1993). Therefore, women who are optimistic tend to cope after surgery by using certain cognitive strategies, which is in turn associated with less distress over time and thus helps them adjust better to the cancer experience than their more pessimistic counterparts, who are prone to use less productive coping strategies such as denial and disengagement.

These findings played a key role in our choice to use cognitive restructuring as a centerpiece of the B-SMART program. As noted previously, cognitive restructuring is used to teach the women to (a) think about the cognitive appraisals they have about their illness and ongoing stressors and then (b) correct any distortions they may be harboring. This process may pave the way toward making their appraisals more positive—the process of positive reframing. In some cases, cognitive restructuring could help some women with breast cancer realize that certain aspects of their lives are simply unchangeable (e.g., the loss of a breast).

They are encouraged to use acceptance as a coping strategy, use other coping strategies to deal with their emotional reactions to this realization (e.g., relaxation for anxiety), and use more direct, problem-focused coping efforts to handle aspects of their life that are more changeable (e.g., investing in personal relationships, seeking out medical information, exploring complementary therapies). As indicated in our empirical work, adopting strategies such as positive reframing and being more accepting may help these women become more optimistic individuals and experience less distress.

RELIGION

■ "Religiosity, Religious Coping, and Distress: A Prospective Study of Catholic and Evangelical Hispanic Women in Treatment for Early Stage Breast Cancer" (Alferi et al., 1999).

Some women rely quite heavily on the use of religion as a coping strategy, especially for coping with stressors from life-threatening diseases. We found evidence that the use of religion as a coping strategy by women at the time that they were diagnosed with early-stage breast cancer prospectively predicted their emotional adjustment in the months after surgery. Interestingly, the ways in which religious coping predicted emotional adjustment varied as a function of their religious affiliation. Evangelical/Protestant women who used religion as a coping strategy reported less distress after surgery, whereas Catholic women who used religion as a coping strategy reported greater distress after surgery. These findings allowed us to begin to address the fact that religious beliefs, as well as sociocultural and ethnic factors, may play a role in the effectiveness of specific coping choices. Therefore, it is critical that psychosocial interventions used to alter coping strategies in patients with breast cancer address personal beliefs and cultural factors—an essential step if the interventions are to improve the patients' emotional adjustment and quality of life. We paid special attention to these factors in the development of the B-SMART program. We have recently completed a Spanish version of the intervention that has been designed to address the ways in which certain coping strategies and stress management techniques (e.g., assertiveness training) might be received by Spanish-speaking women with breast cancer.

SOCIAL SUPPORT

■ "An Exploratory Study of Social Support, Distress, and Disruption Among Low Income Hispanic Women Under Treatment for Early Stage Breast Cancer" (Alferi, Carver, et al., 2001).

Many studies of patients with breast cancer have found that perceived availability of support relates to less distress (Bloom, 1982; Funch & Mettlin, 1982; Nelles, McCaffrey, Blanchard, & Ruckdeschel, 1991; Wortman, 1984; for review, see Helgeson & Cohen, 1996). The type of support most commonly given to patients with breast cancer is emotional (compassion, caring, and concern); instrumental support (advice, transportation, money) is less common (Dunkel-Schetter, 1984; Pistrang & Barker, 1995; E. M. Smith, Redman, Burns, & Sagert, 1986; Wortman, 1984). Indeed, one review concluded that emotional support improves adjustment to breast cancer, but instrumental support does not (Helgeson & Cohen, 1996). However, the latter conclusion is based on very few studies. One study found instrumental support to be unrelated to concurrent depressive symptoms (Primomo, Yates, & Woods, 1990), and another study found that it was related to *more* depressive symptoms (Penninx et al., 1998). On the other hand, some patients have reported that instrumental support is very helpful (Dakof & Taylor, 1990). Thus, it seems premature to assume instrumental support has no role in the emotional well-being of patients with cancer. A separate issue is whether some sources of support are more helpful than others. A third issue concerns whether source and type of support relate to adjustment in ethnic minority women in the same ways that they do in the previously studied, mainly White, individuals.

We examined the relationships between distress and perceived availability of social support in 51 Hispanic women being treated for early-stage breast cancer (Alferi, Carver, et al., 2001). This prospective study measured distress and different types of support (i.e., emotional, instrumental) and sources of support (i.e., spouse, women family members, other family members, friends) before surgery, after surgery, and at 3-, 6-, and 12-month follow-ups. Emotional support before surgery from friends and instrumental support before surgery from the spouse predicted lower distress after surgery (see Table 2.2). Among unmarried women, emotional support after surgery from women in the family predicted less distress at the 3-month follow-up, but instrumental support before surgery from the family predicted higher distress after surgery. We wondered whether distress levels at one point could actually forecast a loss or erosion of social support at a subsequent point. Indeed, distress at several different points after surgery predicted erosion of subsequent support, particularly instrumental support from women in the family. This may be related to the fact that women's social networks tend to burn out during the trying period of breast cancer treatment. In contrast to the effects of distress (and independent of them), illness-related disruption of recreational and social activities at 6 months predicted higher levels of support at 12 months.

These findings were extremely useful in helping us understand the most salient aspects of social support and the ways in which social support can erode over time during cancer treatment among Hispanic women with breast cancer. This information was critical in developing many of the components of the B-SMART intervention, a program that is designed to offer numerous benefits through the provision of support and techniques designed to increase or maintain support in patients' lives. We learned that emotional and instrumental support can be differentially effective based on the origin of the support. Therefore, certain sessions of the B-SMART program provide exercises designed to increase awareness of subtle differences between emotional and instrumental aspects of support. In addition, some sessions of the B-SMART program focus on using emotional coping responses and resources for unchangeable stressors and problem-focused (instrumental) responses and resources for changeable stressors.

Alternative and Complementary Therapy Among Women With Breast Cancer

■ "Factors Predicting the Use of Complementary Therapies in a Multi-Ethnic Sample of Early-Stage Breast Cancer Patients" (Alferi, Antoni, Ironson, Kilbourn, & Carver, 2001).

Where do women with breast cancer tend to seek out support? In the past several years, the popularity and commonsense appeal of cancer support groups and psychosocial counseling for cancer patients and their families has grown substantially. A wide variety of medical patient populations are also becoming more interested in the use of alternative and complementary therapies that purport to offer relief, spiritual support, and, in some cases, cures from medical conditions. Numerous patients diagnosed with cancer have shown an interest in these types of therapy. Some of our work has focused on identifying the prevalence of the use of alternative and complementary therapies among women diagnosed with early-stage breast cancer. A second issue we have explored concerns the demographic, ethnic, medical, and psychosocial characteristics that predict the use of these services. Although we do not classify the B-SMART program as a complementary or an alternative therapy, some women dealing with breast cancer may do so. Thus, by investigating factors associated with the pursuit and use of these therapies, we hoped to gain

Concurrent Correlations Between Distress and Perceived Emotional and Instrumental Support Available From Various Sources at Each Time Point

Type and support		Shorter term				Longer term	
	N	Pre	Post	3 month	*N*	6 month	12 month
Emotional support							
Spouse	22	−.59**	−.66**	−.48**	18	−.57**	−.20
Female family members	44	−.23	−.16	−.13	40	−.09	−.45**
Other family members	42	−.22	−.13	.02	38	−.16	−.15
Friends	48	−.32	−.13	.07	43	−.38**	.05
Instrumental support							
Spouse	23	−.54**	−.41*	−.21	19	−.72**	−.41*
Female family members	44	−.01	−.06	−.00	40	−.14	−.26
Other family members	40	−.16	.13	−.05	37	.04	−.22
Friends	50	−.04	.10	−.14	46	.03	.37**

Note. Longer term *N* is a subset of shorter term *N*. Pre = presurgery; Post = postsurgery. From "An Exploratory Study of Social Support, Distress, and Disruption Among Low-Income Hispanic Women Under Treatment for Early-Stage Breast Cancer," by S. Alferi, C. S. Carver, M. H. Antoni, S. Weiss, and R. Duran, 2001, *Health Psychology, 20*, pp. 41–46. Copyright 2001 by the American Psychological Association. Reprinted with permission.

$*p < .08. **p < .05.$

some insight into factors that might characterize the types of women most likely to seek out the B-SMART program.

We examined the use of complementary treatments and psychological and physical factors that predict their use in a group of multiethnic women, which included numerous Hispanic patients and a smaller subsample of African American patients. The 231 women with early-stage breast cancer (11 stage 0, 135 stage I, and 85 stage II) were recruited through several Miami area hospitals and practices. Use of alternative therapies was assessed by asking, "Have you used any of the following nontraditional, alternative health care services in treating your breast cancer? Acupuncture, herbal medication, meditation/imagery, massage/body therapy, spiritual healing." For the sake of comparison with more "mainstream" therapies, participants were also asked, "Have you used psychotherapy or counseling services to help with the social or emotional aspects of your illness?" and "Have you participated in a breast cancer support group?"

The most frequently used therapies were meditation/imagery, support groups, psychotherapy, and spiritual healing. Support groups were used by a larger proportion of patients who had received a mastectomy (32%) than who had received a lumpectomy (18%). Undergoing psychotherapy was more common among younger than older women; two times more premenopausal women than postmenopausal women reported doing so. Psychotherapy use was also more common among those with higher levels of education. Psychotherapy also related to all measures of distress and concern. Women who reported use of psychotherapy reported higher distress on the POMS and higher scores on the Center for Epidemiologic Survey of Depression (CES–D) than those who did not report using psychotherapy. Women reporting use of psychotherapy also had higher levels of concern on each of three factors of the PCBC and higher levels of sexual disturbance.

Use of healing therapies (e.g., herbal medication, spiritual healing) was more likely among younger women, those receiving chemotherapy, those further along in treatment, those with later stage disease, the employed, certain religious groups, and those who expected to remain free of cancer. We also examined the therapies separately, which yielded a more differentiated picture. Proportionally more African American women (35%) than either Hispanic (12%) or non-Hispanic White (12%) women reported use of herbal therapies. Most women reporting use of massage were also undergoing chemotherapy. They were also more educated than those not using massage and were overall more confident about their disease not recurring.

Use of spiritual healing was strongly related to ethnicity: The majority of African American women in the sample had used spiritual healing, whereas only 16% of Hispanic and 18% of non-Hispanic White women did. The religion of the participants also played a role in whether they used spiritual healing. More of the women endorsing Christian-non-Catholic and "other" religions indicated using spiritual healing than did Catholics or Jews. The use of spiritual healing was also related to undergoing chemotherapy and to later stages of disease. (Of those who used this technique, 55% were in chemotherapy.) Finally, women who reported using spiritual healing were also younger than those who did not.

Use of meditation/imagery also related strongly to menopausal status. The majority of women who reported using meditation/imagery were premenopausal, with 39% of all premenopausal women in the sample having used meditation/imagery. Chemotherapy also related to use of meditation/imagery. (Of all women in chemotherapy, 44% reported that they meditated.) Women who used meditation also had more positive nodes than women who did not. We found that use of healing therapies was not related to pain, pain-related disruptions, or dissatisfaction with medical treatment. As a group, these findings contradict the idea that patients turn to complementary medicine because they are in despair about their chances of survival or dissatisfied with their medical care

(Burstein, Gelber, Guadagnoli, & Weeks, 1999). Rather, the findings suggest that most people who use healing therapies are exploring ways to complement the benefits already being obtained from medical therapies. The idea that the women use healing therapies to explore additional forms of care corresponds with the greater prevalence among younger and more educated women.

These findings helped us identify the women who might be interested in seeking out stress management as a means of dealing with cancer-related concerns and cancer treatments such as chemotherapy. Women seeking out healing therapies such as herbal therapies, massage, spiritual healing, and meditation/imagery may think of them as healthy ways to offset the toxic effects of chemotherapy rather than as alternatives to traditional medical intervention. Women seeking out psychotherapy appear to be younger and more educated but also more distressed than those not seeking these services. Finally, those seeking out support groups seem to have no major differences from those who do not, except that they are more likely to have undergone a mastectomy than a lumpectomy. Because the B-SMART program has several features of these therapies, including meditation/imagery, psychotherapy, and a supportive group environment, we have surmised that our intervention might be particularly in line with the choices made by younger, more educated women with breast cancer, and it might be particularly helpful to those dealing with chemotherapy. The initial evaluations of the B-SMART program were actually conducted with younger women (i.e., younger than age 60 years) who were recovering from surgery and beginning their adjuvant therapy regimen. We are in the process of learning how these techniques can be adjusted so that they are as useful as possible for older, less educated, and more ethnically diverse women dealing with breast cancer. Some of these studies are elaborated in a later section of this chapter.

What are the Effects of CBSM Intervention on Depression and Benefit Finding After a Diagnosis of Breast Cancer?

■ "Cognitive–Behavioral Stress Management Intervention Enhances Optimism and the Sense of Positive Contributions Among Women

Under Treatment for Early-Stage Breast Cancer" (Antoni et al., 2001).

While developing the B-SMART program, we were interested in providing women with distress reduction techniques and strategies for helping them find benefits in the cancer experience (i.e., benefit finding). To monitor distress reduction, we used the CES–D (Radloff, 1977), an index of depressive symptoms experienced by nonpsychiatric samples. To monitor positive changes during the intervention, we created a measure of positive responses to the experience of diagnosis and treatment of breast cancer that we refer to as the Benefit Finding Scale (BFS; see display). This measure taps several different aspects of positive responses, ranging from the social (closer ties to family and friends) to the existential (focusing on one's life priorities, acceptance of life's unchangeable aspects) to enhancement of coping skills. Despite their divergent origins, the 17 items had good internal consistency. Reports of benefit finding (aggregated across items) related to lower levels of distress. Benefit finding scores also related to one of the resiliency/vulnerability factors in this sample—optimism; more optimistic women reported greater benefits.

The study was conducted for 4 years (Antoni et al., 2001) and focused on younger patients with breast cancer. In a supportive group format, the intervention provided training and practice in relaxation, coping, assertiveness, and various stress management skills. The intervention thus taught broad life skills, using the diagnosis and treatment for cancer as the exemplar of a stressor rather than focusing entirely on the cancer experience. The intervention began 4 to 8 weeks after surgery. Women randomized to a comparison group received a 1-day seminar 3 months after treatment (roughly the time the B-SMART intervention groups were ending). All women were assessed before the intervention, at the 3-month point, and again 3 and 9 months later.

Because the women had to attend weekly group meetings for 10 weeks while they were also balancing their adjuvant therapy schedule with job- and family-related responsibilities, we were especially cognizant of participant attendance rates and attrition rates. Of the cohorts assessed to date, we have found a cumulative attrition rate of 12% (equivalent across conditions). Among intervention women, attendance at sessions averaged 89%. Attrition and attendance rates across cohorts were also relatively consistent.

Analyses were conducted on data obtained from 99 women through the 9-month follow-up (Antoni et al., 2001). Analysis of this group revealed several points. First, distress reported was never high, even several weeks after surgery. This is typical of recent data from patients with early-stage breast cancer. (For example, Carver et al., 1993, reported slight elevation in POMS before surgery, which decreased to normal levels by 2

Items Assessing Benefit Finding in Regard to Having Had Breast Cancer

Having had breast cancer . . .

1. has led me to be more accepting of things.
2. has taught me how to adjust to things I cannot change.
3. has helped me take things as they come.
4. has brought my family closer together.
5. has made me more sensitive to family issues.
6. has taught me that everyone has a purpose in life.
7. has shown me that all people need to be loved.
8. has made me realize the importance of planning for my family's future.
9. has made me more aware and concerned for the future of all human beings.
10. has taught me to be patient.
11. has led me to deal better with stress and problems.
12. has led me to meet people who have become some of my best friends.
13. has contributed to my overall emotional and spiritual growth.
14. has helped me become more aware of the love and support available from other people.
15. has helped me realize who my real friends are.
16. has helped me become more focused on priorities, with a deeper sense of purpose in life.
17. has helped me become a stronger person, more able to cope effectively with future life challenges.

Note. From "Cognitive–Behavioral Stress Management Intervention Decreases the Prevalence of Depression and Enhances Benefit Finding Among Women Under Treatment for Early-Stage Breast Cancer," by M. H. Antoni, J. Lehman, K. Kilbourn, A. Boyers, S. Yount, J. Culver, et al., 2001, *Health Psychology, 20,* pp. 20–32. Copyright 2001 by the American Psychological Association. Reprinted with permission.

weeks after surgery and remained at that level at all subsequent measures.) As a result of this "floor effect" on distress, the intervention resulted in no additional distress reduction. However, we did note that when about 25% of the women began the study, they had clinically elevated depression scores (i.e., a CES–D score of greater than 16). During the course of the study, we found that the scores of more than half of these women who were assigned to the B-SMART program decreased to a point that they were no longer considered clinically depressed, whereas those in the control condition (at a 9-month follow-up) did not show this pattern (Antoni et al., 2001; see Figure 2.1).

Numerous other positive changes were also observed in women assigned to the B-SMART intervention. The intervention and control groups did not differ on the benefit-finding measure immediately after surgery. However, by the time the 10-week B-SMART program was completed,

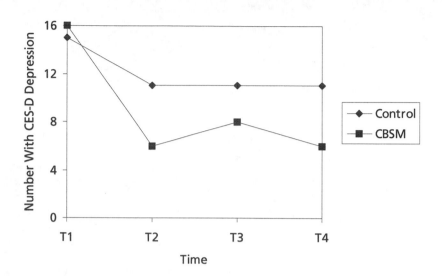

Number of patients with breast cancer scoring higher than the cutoff for depression (CES–D scores greater than 16) in CBSM intervention vs. control conditions at the beginning of the intervention (T1), after the intervention (T2), at the 3-month follow-up (T3), and at the 9-month follow-up (T4).

the women in the B-SMART group had significantly higher benefit-finding scores, whereas the control group's score was virtually unchanged. This score was still higher at the 3- and 9-month follow-ups as well. The extent of benefit finding related to the coping response of positive reframing at the beginning of the study, after the intervention, and at the 3-month follow-up; benefit finding was inversely related to denial coping after the intervention. These findings suggest that women participating in B-SMART find more benefits in the cancer experience, and those who use more positive reframing (a major focus of CBSM) and less denial have the most improvements in benefit finding at the follow-ups.

We also found that women assigned to B-SMART became significantly more optimistic, whereas no such changes were observed in control women. This suggests that the intervention may have helped the women to begin changing their outlook on different aspects of their lives. Paralleling this pattern after the intervention were reports that B-SMART participants were examining and expressing their feelings more (as measured by the Emotional Processing Scales; Stanton et al., 2000); those in the control condition were not. Thus, the intervention was effective in prompting participants to examine and express their feelings, another major aim of the B-SMART program. One of the most interesting findings of this study was that women who were initially classified as pessimists on the basis of their scores on the LOT–R were the women who had the greatest increases in benefit finding scores during the B-SMART intervention (see Figure 2.2, *top panel*). Thus, the B-SMART program may be particularly beneficial to women with the most negative outlooks during their breast cancer treatment.

In sum, the pattern of findings for positive responses in this study fits with the observation noted previously—many patients with cancer report that having the disease has had positive consequences. However, the program's effects go beyond this finding. It appears that the B-SMART program successfully creates a stronger sense of the positive in its participants. If the positive outlook then has a positive effect on physical responses, its impact on quality of life—physical as well as psychological—may be substantial. This possibility is an ongoing part of our research program. The disposition to be optimistic is a very stable personality trait (Scheier & Carver, 1992), and this is the first time of which we are aware that an intervention of this sort has raised dispositional optimism scores. Because optimism has been related to better physical health in various populations (Scheier & Carver, 1992), CBSM-based programs such as B-SMART may offer benefits for people dealing with other chronic medical difficulties.

What Types of Physiological Changes Occur During the B-SMART Program?

▪ "Cognitive–Behavioral Stress Management Reduces Serum Cortisol by Enhancing Positive Contributions Among Women Being Treated for Early Stage Breast Cancer" (D. Cruess, Antoni, McGregor, et. al., 2000).

▪ "Cognitive Behavioral Stress Management Effects on Testosterone and Positive Growth in Women With Early-Stage Breast Cancer" (Cruess, Antoni, McGregor, et al., 2001).

▪ "Adjustment to Breast Cancer: The Psychobiological Effects of Psychosocial Interventions" (van der Pompe, Antoni, Visser, & Garssen, 1996).

▪ "Effectiveness of a Short-Term Group Psychotherapy Program on Endocrine and Immune Function in Breast Cancer Patients" (van der Pompe, Duivenvoorden, et al., 1997).

▪ "The Relations of Plasma ACTH and Cortisol Levels With the Distribution and Function of Peripheral Blood Cells in Response to a

FIGURE 2.2

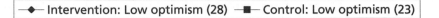

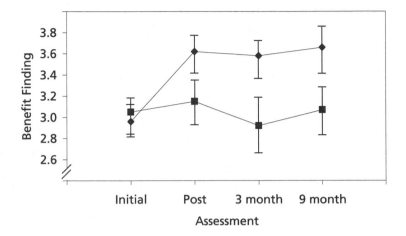

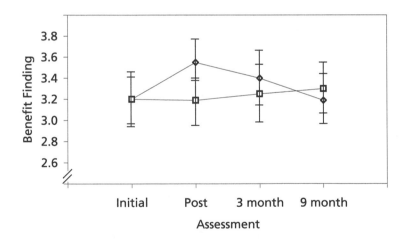

Benefit finding among patients with early-stage breast cancer in the intervention and control conditions; participants were either relatively low in initial optimism *(top panel)* or relatively high in initial optimism *(bottom panel)*. Benefit finding was reported at the initial, posttreatment, 3-month follow-up, and 9-month follow-up assessments. (Group *n*s are shown in parentheses.) From "Cognitive–Behavioral Stress Management Intervention Decreases the Prevalence of Depression and Enhances Benefit Finding Among Women Under Treatment for Early-Stage Breast cancer," by M. H. Antoni, J. Lehman, K. Kilbourn, A. Boyers, S. Yount, J. Culver, et al., 2001, *Health Psychology, 20,* pp. 20–32. Copyright 2001 by the American Psychological Association. Adapted with permission.

Behavioral Challenge in Breast Cancer" (van der Pompe, Antoni, & Heijnen, 1997).

▌ "Effects of Cognitive–Behavioral Stress Management on Immune Function and Positive Contributions in Women With Early-Stage Breast Cancer" (McGregor et al., 2000).

ENDOCRINE–IMMUNE RELATIONSHIPS IN PATIENTS WITH BREAST CANCER

One study that conducted work in the Netherlands examined mechanisms by which stress and a psychosocial intervention of similar intensity to the B-SMART program might relate to immune system functioning in patients with early- to mid-stage breast cancer (stages I through III) and those with metastatic disease (stage IV). Compared with healthy women, patients with breast cancer had higher plasma cortisol levels and smaller lymphocyte proliferative responses to challenge and related lymphocyte counts (CD4+ T cells) at baseline and across a standardized behavioral challenge (van der Pompe, Antoni, & Heijnen, 1997, 1998). Higher cortisol concentrations related to less lymphocyte proliferation in both the stage I through III group and the stage IV group. This suggests that chronically elevated levels of cortisol may be partially responsible for decrements in lymphocyte number and proliferation in these patients. Interestingly, despite elevations in cortisol level and lower proliferative responses, these women did not differ from age-matched healthy control women in distress levels. This suggests that the endocrine and immune status were independent of distress processes. Our work actually indicates that other psychological processes—emotional expression and benefit finding—may be more influential on cortisol levels and immune functioning in women with breast cancer (e.g., D. Cruess, Antoni, McGregor, et al., 2000; McGregor et al., 2000).

In another set of projects, which were conducted in Holland, we tested the effects of a 13-week group therapy program (compared with a wait-list control group) on one of these psychological processes—emotional expression—among Dutch women with stages I, II, III, or IV breast cancer. The intervention encouraged women to express their emotions through self-disclosure, modify their coping strategies, and change their life perspective to draw more meaning from the cancer experience (van der Pompe, Duivenvoorden, et al., 1997). Like the B-SMART intervention, this intervention had no effect on distress reduction compared with control women, but the intervention group was more emotionally expressive after treatment (as shown by reductions in the Emotions-in subscale of the Emotional Expression Scale; Watson & Greer, 1983). We did not collect information on benefit finding, but it is possible that emotional expression paved the way for positive results like it seemed to in the B-SMART program (Antoni et al., 2001). The intervention group also had lower levels of plasma cortisol after treatment than did the control group (van der Pompe, Duivenvoorden, et al., 1997).

Finally, we examined how the 13-week intervention affected the immune systems of the Dutch women. To test the ability of the intervention to buffer stress-induced changes in the immune system, we brought the women to a laboratory and used a stress reactivity paradigm. In this experiment, we first exposed each woman to a laboratory challenge wherein they were required to give a stressful evaluative speech while being videotaped. We recorded cardiovascular responses (e.g., systolic and diastolic blood pressure) and drew five blood samples during the stress reactivity task. After the women completed this session, they were randomized to either the 13-week intervention or a 13-week waiting period. At the end of this period, they returned to the laboratory and completed a different challenge, during which physiological parameters were again collected. We were trying to determine whether women in the intervention maintained better immune system functioning during the stressful experience. To monitor the immune system, we measured (among other things) natural killer (NK) cell counts and natural killer cell cytotoxicity (NKCC) from each blood sample collected. Thus, we collected five measurements during an evaluative speech task conducted before and after the intervention and compared changes in proliferation between intervention and control participants. We found that women in the intervention group showed smaller stress-induced changes in NK cell counts and NKCC compared with those in the control group (van der Pompe et al., 2001). Importantly, women who showed the largest increase in emotional expression showed the smallest stress-induced immune changes over this period. These findings suggest that the intervention may have buffered the effects of stress on immune functioning by increasing emotional expression. As noted, emotional expression may have facilitated positive responses—likewise, the experience of disclosing emotions may have influenced immune system functioning directly (Esterling et al., 1994; Pennebaker, Kiecolt-Glaser, & Glaser, 1988; Petrie, Booth, Pennebaker, Davidson, & Thomas, 1995). These findings provide preliminary justification for further studies of mechanisms underlying intervention effects on immune system changes through psychological processes. In parallel with this work, we also examined the effects of our B-SMART program on similar physiological parameters among American women.

EFFECTS OF B-SMART ON CORTISOL PRODUCTION IN WOMEN WITH BREAST CANCER

We conducted analyses of cortisol levels using blood samples taken from a subset of 34 women participating in the evaluation studies of the B-SMART program (D. Cruess, Antoni, McGregor, et al., 2000). Analysis of these women (24 intervention, 10 control) revealed that although there was no group difference before intervention, intervention participants had lower levels of cortisol after B-SMART than control participants (see Figure 2.3). Greater reductions in cortisol were also significantly related to changes in benefit finding during the 10-week intervention period.

Furthermore, path analysis suggested that the effect of the intervention on cortisol change was mediated by positive changes induced by the intervention (see Figure 2.4). As shown in the figure, although the intervention appeared to decrease cortisol and increase benefit finding, including benefit finding in the regression equation used to predict cortisol levels after treatment appeared to explain most of the effects of B-SMART on cortisol levels (D. Cruess, Antoni, McGregor, et al., 2000). These findings were the same after controlling for age, estradiol, and chemotherapy status. This pattern indicates that the intervention had an impact on an aspect of the physiological response (as measured by cortisol levels in the

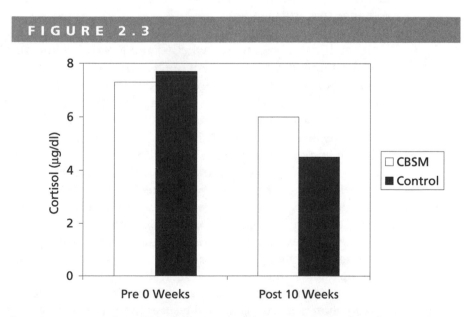

FIGURE 2.3

Pretreatment and posttreatment mean plasma cortisol values for patients with breast cancer in CBSM vs. control conditions.

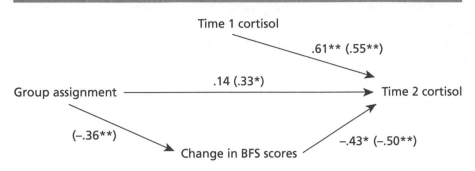

FIGURE 2.4

Path model testing the mediating effect of changes in BFS scores on the relationship between group assignment (CBSM vs. control) and serum cortisol changes. Simple associations are shown in parentheses, and standardized regression coefficients from the full model are shown outside parentheses ($*p < .05$. $**p < .01$). From "Cognitive-Behavioral Stress Management Reduces Serum Cortisol by Enhancing Benefit Finding Among Women Being Treated for Early Stage Breast Cancer," by D. G. Cruess, M. H. Antoni, B. A. McGregor, K. M. Kilbourn, A. E. Boyers, S. M. Alferi, et al., 2001, *Psychosomatic Medicine, 62*, pp. 304–308. Copyright 2000 by the American Psychosomatic Society. Adapted with permission.

peripheral blood). Furthermore, it prompted a positive psychological change in participants.

By studying changes in serum testosterone levels during the course of the study, we also explored whether the B-SMART intervention affected sex hormone function. As mentioned in chapter 1, changes in levels of sex hormones such as testosterone may increase the risk of breast cancer in women (Berrino et al., 1996) and may predict recurrence after treatment (Cruess, Antoni, McGregor, et al., 2001). Specifically, alterations in testosterone level may influence the progression of breast cancer by changing the binding of testosterone to cancer cells, decreasing intratissue aromatization of testosterone to estradiol and reducing stimulation of epithelial growth factor by testosterone (Secreto & Zumoff, 1994). We found significant decreases in total and free testosterone in the women assigned to B-SMART and no changes in control women (Cruess, Antoni, McGregor, et al., 2001). These findings were the same after controlling for differences in alcohol use, changes in estradiol levels, cigarette smoking, and chemotherapy status. Interestingly, women showing the greatest increases in benefit finding showed the greatest reductions in testosterone (see Figure 2.5). In addition, reductions in total testosterone were strongly associated with decreases in cortisol during the intervention period, suggesting the possibility that the two hormones, one a stress hormone (cortisol) and one a sex hormone (testosterone), may interact in women with breast cancer.

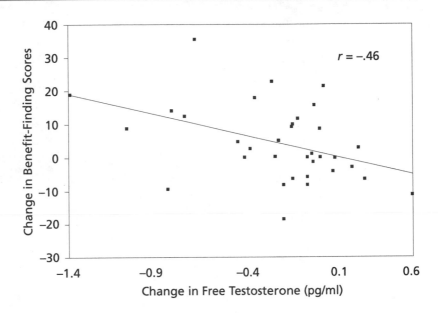

Bivariate distribution for T1–T2 serum free testosterone change scores and benefit finding change scores.

EFFECTS OF B-SMART ON IMMUNE STATUS IN WOMEN WITH BREAST CANCER

Data from 34 women participating in the B-SMART evaluation studies who had blood samples drawn at the beginning of the study and at the 3-month follow-up were also analyzed for the effects of the B-SMART intervention over time. These assays focused specifically on lymphocyte proliferative responses to challenge and Th1 cytokine (interleukin-2 [IL-2]) and Th2 cytokine (IL-4) production from lymphocytes in response to this challenge. Psychological measures included measures that had been shown (in the larger sample) to be affected by the B-SMART intervention and measures correlated with psychosocial changes brought about by the intervention. Measures included the BFS, the Life Orientation Test (LOT; Carver & Scheier, 1990), our optimism measure, the total score for the Social Support Provisions Scale (SPS; Cutrona & Russell, 1987), and the Positive Reframing and Behavioral Disengagement subscales of the COPE.

At the beginning of the study, greater lymphocyte proliferation was associated with more total social support provisions, more optimism, greater use of positive reframing, and less use of behavioral disengagement as coping strategies. Higher cortisol levels were associated with lower proliferation, less IL-2 production, and more IL-4 production. This pat-

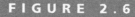

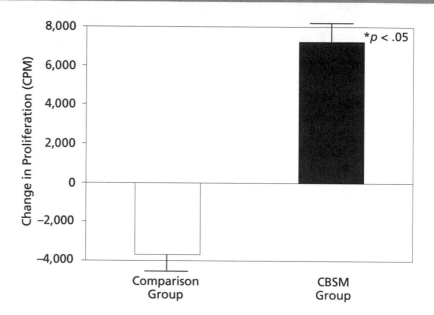

Mean change in proliferative response (counts per minute, CPM) to anti-CD3 from preintervention to 3-month follow-up in patients with breast cancer assigned to the control condition or the CBSM intervention condition.

tern of results suggests that psychosocial factors such as use of positive reframing coping, optimism, and perceived social support (which are targets of the B-SMART program) and lower levels of cortisol are associated greater immune responses to challenge, more production of Th1 cytokines, and less production of Th2 cytokines, a pattern that may promote optimal surveillance of cancer cells.

In additional tests of this sample of 34 women, our emphasis was on the direct effects of B-SMART on changes observable up to 3 months after the intervention. By this point, most participants have completed their chemotherapy and radiation regimen, thus their immune responses are less likely to be influenced by adjuvant therapy. We found a Group × Time interaction on proliferation, with women in B-SMART showing an increase and control women showing a decrease (see Figure 2.6). We also found that increases in benefit finding during the period of the intervention were associated with greater increases in lymphocyte proliferation from the initial measure to the 3-month follow-up (see Figure 2.7; McGregor et al., 2000). Greater decreases in avoidance responses during the initial intervention period also related to greater increase in proliferation at 3-month follow-up. Therefore, although still preliminary, these findings suggest that women assigned to B-SMART had improvements

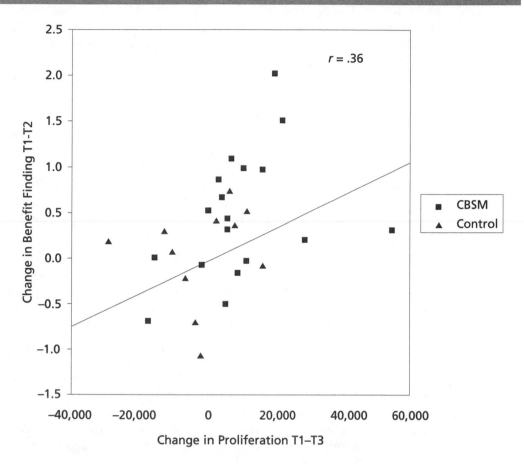

Correlation between change in proliferative response to anti-CD3 (counts per minute) and change in benefit finding among patients with breast cancer assigned to the CBSM intervention or the control condition. T1 = preintervention; T2 = postintervention; T3 = 3-month follow-up.

in immune status, and those revealing the greatest psychological growth or increases in benefit finding experienced the greatest decreases in cortisol and greatest increases in immune status.

Conclusion and Ongoing Investigations

The conceptual base that guides our work is as follows: We believe personality and social context predispose some people to be more responsive to problems inherent in the diagnosis and treatment of breast cancer. The relevant factors may be thought of as indicators of vulnerability or resilience. The immediate responses prompted by the variables represent a set of mediators, including confrontation of concerns aroused by the diagnosis, cognitive coping reaction, perceived skill at using stress management techniques, and perceived social provisions. These mediators help determine the levels of the outcome variables: positive adaptations in emotional, attitudinal, interpersonal, and behavioral health spheres; negative adaptations such as emotional distress, physical changes, social disengagement, and poor psychosexual adjustment; and changes in the immune system and physical health outcomes.

The B-SMART program is largely designed to target mediating variables for change. Although one goal is to modify vulnerability variables, we also tried to induce a greater sense of optimism and a more positive outlook regarding recurrence. One of the chief and recurring themes of our intervention is the importance of raising awareness of ongoing challenges and awareness of participants' immediate responses (cognitive appraisals) to these challenges. Once they raise their awareness, especially in the first third of the intervention, women are taught methods to change their cognitive appraisals and avoid catastrophic thinking. As more rational appraisals of disease outcomes evolve, the intervention encourages the women to continually confront their cancer-related concerns. Continued confrontation could lead to greater acceptance and assimilation of the diagnosis. It seems beneficial to encourage participants to retain and enhance their levels of social integration, a process that is facilitated by the group format and explicit training in interpersonal skills (anger management, assertiveness training) designed to enhance the quality of relationships (e.g., through improved communication and decreased conflict).

Thus, we designed the B-SMART intervention to achieve positive outcomes by fostering confidence in the future (with respect to recurrence and life in general), by altering coping responses (increasing acceptance of the situation and reducing denial and avoidance coping), by increasing perceived skill at using stress management techniques, by increasing the sense of support from others, by enhancing self-concept, and by fostering an attitude of continuing engagement with life. The intervention may help participants achieve these goals by teaching behavioral and cognitive strategies and providing them the opportunity to role-play, using coping strategies in situations reflecting their most important concerns.

The theoretical model underlying the effects of CBSM interventions such as B-SMART on psychological adjustment and physical health outcomes in patients with breast cancer is outlined in Figure 2.8. According to this model, the B-SMART intervention immediately addresses a series of intervention targets, which in turn can change quality-of-life variables, positive and negative health behaviors, immune status, and levels

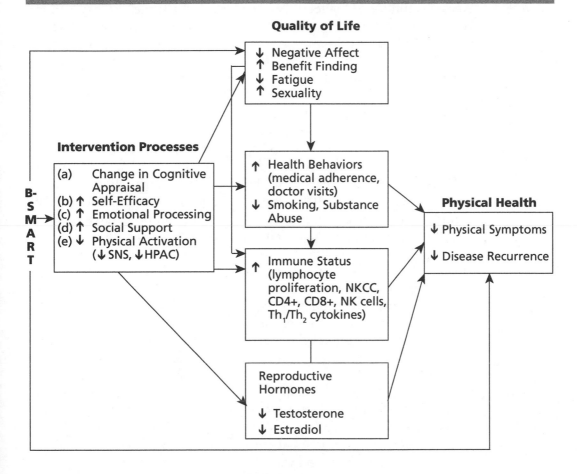

FIGURE 2.8

Theoretical model for effects of B-SMART intervention for women with breast cancer.

of reproductive hormones. These changes are in turn hypothesized to predict longer term changes in physical health. Among the improvements hypothesized to occur during B-SMART are increases in rational cognitive appraisals of stressors, increases in self-efficacy, increases in emotional processing (focusing on and expressing emotions), increases in perceived social support, and decreases in the production of sympathetic nervous system hormones such as epinephrine and norepinephrine and HPAC hormones such as cortisol. Among the hypothesized changes in quality of life are decreases in negative affect and fatigue and increases in benefit finding and sexuality. The B-SMART program is also hypothesized to increase positive behaviors such as medical adherence, attendance at follow-up appointments, and sleeping well. In addition, the program should decrease negative health behaviors such as smoking and substance use. Among the immunological measures, we hypothesize that the B-

SMART program will increase CD4+ and CD8+ lymphocyte counts, increase lymphocyte proliferative responses to challenge, increase NK cell counts and NKCC, increase production of Th1 cytokines, and decrease production of Th2 cytokines. Based on our preliminary studies, we are hypothesizing that this intervention may also decrease levels of the sex hormones testosterone and estradiol. Finally, we hypothesize that women in the B-SMART intervention will have better physical health outcomes, including less physical symptoms (e.g., infectious disease symptoms) and a lower incidence of disease recurrence.

In the past decade, our group has carried out numerous intervention studies of patients who are dealing with breast cancer by using the B-SMART program or other CBSM-based interventions tailored to other medical diseases such as HIV infection. The most consistent findings with regard to the psychological effects of the interventions have been (a) decreases in distress and depressed affect, (b) decreases in the use of avoidance and denial as coping strategies, (c) increases in the use of acceptance and positive reframing strategies, (d) increases or maintenance of social support, and (e) increases in a sense of optimism and benefit finding in the cancer experience. Many of these psychological changes have been accompanied by alterations in adrenal stress hormones such as cortisol and catecholamines (e.g., norepinephrine), sex hormones such as testosterone, and immune system status in men with HIV infection (Antoni, Cruess, Cruess, et al., 2000; Antoni, Cruess, Wagner, et al., 2000; Cruess, Antoni, Schneiderman, et al., 2000) and women with breast cancer (D. Cruess, Antoni, McGregor, et al., 2000; McGregor et al., 2000). What remains to be determined is whether these psychological and physiological changes predict optimal physical health status and decreased disease recurrence in these individuals. The results of these studies should be available in the next few years.

To date, validation of the B-SMART program has demonstrated its efficacy in decreasing the prevalence of moderate depression and increasing positive psychological factors such as general optimism and benefit finding among women with early-stage breast cancer who are undergoing initial treatment. The B-SMART program has also been shown to be capable of reducing adrenal stress hormones such as cortisol and sex hormones such as testosterone to normal concentration ranges, which may improve the physical health of women with breast cancer. In addition to normalizing these hormonal levels, the intervention also appeared to increase the ability of the women's lymphocytes to proliferate in response to antigen challenge. Interestingly, the women who changed the most psychologically during the B-SMART program (e.g., increased benefit finding) also had the largest hormonal decreases during the 10-week intervention period and the greatest levels of lymphocyte proliferation at the 3-month follow-up.

Although these findings are consistent with our theoretical model, it is important to remember that they are preliminary, are based on small samples of women studied shortly after surgery when adjuvant therapy has just begun, and include only a limited number of relevant psychological and physiological indicators. Most importantly, these findings do not establish any evidence for physical health changes resulting from the B-SMART program. The validation findings reported herein should be viewed as a first step in establishing the efficacy of this program.

The next steps are already under way. Aided by funding from the National Cancer Institute, we are now in the process of testing the effects of the B-SMART program in larger samples of women at different stages of breast cancer disease and treatment using a wider array of psychological and physiological readouts. This information is being collected after longer follow-up periods, allowing us to track the effects of B-SMART on physical health outcomes such as disease recurrence and survival. In one study, we are testing the effects of the intervention on disease recurrence and survival among women who completed the B-SMART program (vs. control women) as long as 8 years ago. In this study, we are evaluating survival and disease status and quality of life of survivors in the years after treatment completion. In a second study, women with stages I, II, or III breast cancer are being randomized to B-SMART (or a control condition) approximately 4 to 8 weeks after surgery but before adjuvant therapy has begun and are assessed 3 and 9 months after the 10-week intervention with an extensive panel of immunological parameters (lymphocyte proliferative response, NKCC, Th1 and Th2 cytokine levels) and psychosocial measures (mood, quality of life, benefit finding). The women are then tracked for up to 5 years for quality-of-life changes and signs of recurrence. In a third study, we are testing similar effects in Spanish-speaking women who are participating in a Spanish-language translation of the B-SMART program. In a fourth study, women with stages I, II, or III breast cancer are being randomized to B-SMART (or control) groups 3 months to 1 year after they have completed all of their adjuvant therapy. These women are followed intensively for 15 months and then monitored for a similar 5-year period for quality of life and signs of disease recurrence.

Throughout these different clinical trials, we will examine hypothesized mediators—the active ingredients of the intervention that may be responsible for its effects on quality of life and health outcomes. Possible mediators include changes in relaxation and stress management skills, coping, social support, and emotional expression. We will also examine how theorized demographic (age, ethnicity, socioeconomic status, education), medical (stage), and personality (optimism) factors moderate the effects of the B-SMART program. In so doing, we hope to be able to make recommendations for best adapting this intervention for the individual needs of women dealing with breast cancer.

Details of the B-SMART Program

3

This chapter presents the rationale underlying the development of the B-SMART program and several topics that are useful for implementing the program among women with breast cancer. This section includes

■ the essential domains covered in the program
■ a description of the aims, strategies, and techniques that make up the program
■ a description of the format for running the weekly group sessions
■ an outline of the 10 weekly cognitive–behavioral stress management (CBSM) sessions and their accompanying 10 weekly relaxation session components
■ a description of the materials used for implementing the intervention
■ methods that can be used for selecting, training, and supervising group leaders

Essentials of the B-SMART Program

STRESS MANAGEMENT AND RELAXATION TRAINING

We chose group-based CBSM as a general treatment strategy underlying the B-SMART program. What's in a name? *SMART* (stress management and relaxation training) refers to the stress management techniques and relaxation and imagery exercises that are designed to facilitate participants' efforts to cope with breast cancer and the challenges of daily life. These stress management techniques are designed to increase participants' awareness of their stress response processes and to teach them new ways to think about and act on stressful demands. Some of these techniques focus more on thought patterns and emotional responses, whereas others focus on the ways participants cope and behave in response to stressful events. Still others focus on the ways participants interact with others in interpersonal exchanges and relationships. In addition to learning stress management techniques each week, participants also learn relaxation exercises designed to decrease bodily tension and other physical effects of stress. Some of these exercises teach participants systematically to reduce tension throughout all of their major muscle groups, whereas others teach the participants ways to use mental imagery to bring about a total state of relaxation. The format of B-SMART is a group-experienced therapeutic intervention. This format provides a supportive and collegial environment that should facilitate the learning of new stress-reducing techniques and serve as a place to share current frustrations, inspiration, and ideas with other people who are dealing with similar life circumstances.

The initial impetus for this work came from another study in which we tried to determine whether we could intervene behaviorally to buffer the psychological impact of being diagnosed with an HIV infection (Antoni et al., 1991) and facilitate the people's ability to cope with living with the infection (Antoni, 1997; Lutgendorf et al., 1997, 1998). We believed that several different strategies used in the initial intervention might have been effective in the context of HIV-1 notification. Previously studied interventions with medical patients have tended to focus on either the emotional or cathartic release of pent-up feelings (Pennebaker et. al., 1988; Spiegel, Bloom, Kraemer, & Gottheil, 1989), restructuring maladaptive cognitive appraisals (Beck & Emery, 1979; Burns, 1981), or learning techniques to enhance bodily relaxation (Surwit, Pilon, & Fenton, 1978). Because our initial goal was to offset, or buffer, the acute impact of receiving an HIV-1 diagnosis and facilitate the initial adjustment to the diagnosis, we focused our efforts on stress management techniques. Interventions that focus on stress management have typically used techniques such as cognitive restructuring to increase awareness of how cognitive appraisals about stressors might affect emotions and progressive muscle relaxation (PMR) to reduce anxiety responses to stressful events. We decided that these techniques were equally appropriate for other medical diagnoses including breast cancer. Of course, we were also aware that an intervention initially designed for gay men who were finding out that they were infected with HIV might not readily translate into a form that would be equally effective for women being diagnosed with breast cancer. These target populations differ in many ways including in gender. We thought about which portions of our intervention would have to be tailored to be the most effective for women. We first conducted a series of focus groups with women infected with HIV to learn about their greatest needs, the sorts of coping strategies they were using, and their interpersonal resources. We tailored the intervention accordingly and for numerous years have been using this form of the intervention with women infected with HIV. Because women dealing with breast cancer are coping with a different sort of disease, we addressed the issue of how the intervention would have to be tailored to them as well. Based on a study conducted with hundreds of women dealing with early-stage breast cancer, we learned their greatest concerns, the most effective coping strategies that they used, and how maintaining a positive outlook and adequate social support levels buffered them from persisting distress levels after surgery. We then focused the sessions of the B-SMART intervention on a specific set of intervention targets and used a group-based format.

In our intervention for women dealing with breast cancer, we wanted to use a set of cognitive–behavioral techniques that were standardized, replicable, and portable and had been associated with changes in emotional status (e.g., distress) and physiological functions (e.g., endocrine and immune systems) in prior work. Kiecolt-Glaser and colleagues studied the effects of relaxation training in nursing home residents and medical students. For the nursing home residents, relaxation training was associated with increases in certain indexes of immune functioning (Kiecolt-Glaser, Glaser, & Williger, 1985). Among the medical students, relaxation training seemed to buffer the impact of taking a medical school examination (Kiecolt-Glaser et al., 1986). Specifically, they found that control group students who took the examination had substantial increases in distress and immune decrements, whereas those who were in the relaxation group had much smaller immunological decreases and lower distress levels.

We considered these intervention-associated changes to be a result of modifications of the chronic stress (and stress-related biological changes) faced by the nursing home group and insulation against the students' acute stress. Because both of the groups were generally healthy, little was known about the potential health benefits of offering these types of interventions to stressed people who had medical problems. We extrapolated that relaxation training (and perhaps other stress-reducing techniques) might modify the psychological and physiological effects of stressful events (e.g., receiving a diagnosis, dealing with surgery and adjuvant therapy) in patients with breast cancer, and these modifications would affect the course of the disease. We reasoned that by increasing patients' sense of control and self-efficacy and modifying their self-concept, they might experience less anxiety, depression, and self-isolation. We speculated that these psychological changes might affect the nervous system, which could change the peripheral levels of some immune-modulating hormones (e.g., cortisol). If one could modulate the surveillance capabilities of the immune system (e.g., which would be reflected in increased natural killer cell cytotoxicity [NKCC]) by reducing distress and stress-associated immunomodulatory hormone elevations, then an individual's disease might progress more slowly and perhaps respond better to medical treatment. We developed the B-SMART intervention program as one means of modulating psychological distress levels and accompanying stress-associated hormonal dysregulation in women diagnosed with breast cancer.

In summary, our general model is of breast cancer as a chronic disease, the course of which may be affected by the efficacy of certain immune system components. Factors such as psychosocial and behavioral stressors, which are capable of modulating the immune system, might contribute to immunological decrements, with subsequent complications manifesting as infections and longer term effects such as disease recurrence, metastasis, or death. Behavioral interventions designed to modify the impact of stressors might help these individuals to avoid extreme perturbations of hormonal regulatory systems with less subsequent impact on the immune system and possibly their health. However, our main focus was to decrease distress, increase self-efficacy, improve coping skills, promote feelings of connectedness, and generally improve quality of life.

CHOOSING TREATMENT COMPONENTS

The chief mission of the B-SMART intervention program was to reduce the distress, depression, and maladaptive behaviors that may accompany the diagnosis and treatment for breast cancer and to make patients aware of any beneficial experiences they might have during this period. We had two general questions to answer during the development of this intervention: (a) What are the essential targets of the intervention? (b) Which format would be optimal for addressing these targets?

Intervention Targets

We proposed that CBSM strategies would improve patients' self-efficacy, optimistic outlook, perceptions of social support, and adaptive coping strategies. Receiving a diagnosis of breast cancer and trying to handle the uncertainty of disease progression and relapse can make patients feel that they have lost personal control and result in affective disturbances. Self-efficacy (i.e., beliefs about one's ability to meet situational demands) is known to influence effort, perseverance, personal choices, thought patterns, depression, and perceptions of stress (Bandura, 1986), all of which are salient to people coping with breast cancer. Belief in the ability to manage stressors and change health behaviors may be undermined by a pessimistic attitude, an inability to cope with negative emotions, social isolation, and interpersonal conflict. Cognitive–behavioral techniques (e.g., cognitive restructuring) may modulate self-efficacy, modify attitudes, enhance coping, and improve social support, thereby offering psycho-logical benefits for such individuals. We have hypothesized that cogni-tive restructuring (Beck & Emery, 1979), coping skills training (Folkman et al., 1991), and anger management and assertiveness training (Hersen, Eisler, & Miller, 1973) are viable means for women with breast cancer to accomplish these goals. These techniques may enhance psychological functioning in stressed individuals by (a) increasing perceptions of self-efficacy, personal control, and mastery (Fishman & Loscalzo, 1987); (b) changing maladaptive cognitive distortions (A. D. Simons, Garfield, & Murphy, 1984); (c) modifying stressor appraisals and revealing available coping responses (Turk, Holzman, & Kerns, 1986); (d) decreasing the sense of hopelessness (Rush, Beck, Kovacs, Weissenburger, & Hollon, 1982); and (e) increasing the availability and use of social support net-works (Vachon, Lyall, Rogers, Freedman-Letofsky, & Freeman, 1980). This intervention is tailored to address the issues of loss of personal con-trol, coping demands, social isolation, and depression—all salient for women dealing with breast cancer. Therefore, the B-SMART program may enhance well-being in affective, cognitive, and social spheres of func-tioning on one hand while arming patients with several prophylactic stress buffers on the other.

Intervention Format: The Importance of a Supportive Group Environment

Psychosocial interventions conducted in the context of a supportive group environment may provide a sense of universality, allow individuals with breast cancer to express their feelings, and help them learn about suc-cessful styles of coping used by other group members (Spiegel, Bloom, & Yalom, 1981; Yalom & Greaves, 1977). Group interventions that provide the opportunity for patients with breast cancer to interact and help one another may facilitate coping with the disease and other concerns. In addition to enhancing social support, group psychosocial interventions should build *cognitive and interpersonal skills* needed to deal with stressful encounters. In sum, multimodal stress management interventions that improve cognitive and social/interpersonal coping strategies may be es-pecially useful in reducing *distress* and *depression* and increasing *adjust-ment to the diagnosis and treatment* among women with breast cancer. When such an intervention is conducted in a group format, it provides information, teaches anxiety reduction skills, allows individuals to vent their feelings and frustrations, and builds cognitive and interpersonal coping skills in a supportive group environment.

Intervention Aims, Strategies, and Techniques

The primary aims of the B-SMART program are

- to increase personal awareness by providing information about sources of stress, the nature of human stress responses, and different coping strategies used to deal with stressors
- to teach anxiety reduction skills such as PMR and relaxing imagery techniques
- to modify maladaptive cognitive appraisals using cognitive restructuring
- to enhance cognitive, behavioral, and interpersonal coping skills through coping-skills training, assertion training, and anger management techniques
- to provide a supportive group environment and increase use of social support

To achieve the five aims of the B-SMART program, we use general strategies and specific techniques that are introduced in the 10 weekly group sessions that constitute the program. The facets of the program are summarized in Table 3.1.

AIM 1: INCREASING AWARENESS

The B-SMART program incorporates the most straightforward cognitive–behavioral strategies and accompanying techniques available for accomplishing its five goals. One central feature of the program is the importance of becoming more aware of the components of the stress response. In fact, each of the 10 sessions begins with a section explicitly devoted to building participants' awareness of some aspect of the stress response process.

At the beginning of each session, we attempt to increase awareness by providing information in the form of a didactic lesson that is followed immediately by a group exercise. These exercises include written self-monitoring for daily stressors, conducting body scans, identifying and labeling cognitive appraisals of stressful events, identifying coping responses to stressful events, and imagining threatening and pleasant in-

TABLE 3.1

B-SMART Aims, Strategies, and Techniques

Aims	Strategies	Techniques
Increase awareness of stress responses.	Provide information (i.e., on stress responses); provide in-session experiences.	Didactic and written information, self-monitoring exercises
Teach anxiety reduction skills.	Provide relaxation training.	PMR, guided imagery, autogenics, deep breathing exercises
Modify cognitive appraisals.	Teach CBSM techniques.	Cognitive restructuring, rational thought replacement
Build coping skills and increase emotional expressiveness.	Provide cognitive, behavioral, and interpersonal skills training; facilitate disclosures.	Coping skills training, assertion training, anger management
Reduce social isolation.	Build social support network.	Group support, raising awareness of social network

terpersonal exchanges. These exercises are conducted during the session and are included in homework assignments. For example, participants keep a diary of their daily stress levels and relaxation exercise practice throughout the entire 10 weeks of the program.

AIM 2: TEACHING ANXIETY REDUCTION SKILLS

The second major aim of the program is to teach participants ways to reduce anxiety, tension, and other forms of stress responses. These skills help participants achieve a sense of mastery over some of the many stressful circumstances in their lives. Moreover, by decreasing the intensity of acute emotional or somatic stress responses, participants can better use some of the cognitive, behavioral, and interpersonal skills they are learning to prevent stress responses from multiplying and a sense of helplessness from developing. This may in turn reduce the likelihood of participants becoming depressed or using less healthy coping strategies such as consuming excessive amounts of alcohol or using drugs.

The primary strategies that we use to achieve this goal are relaxation and imagery. In the 10 weekly sessions, we teach participants techniques such as PMR, deep breathing, autogenics, and meditation. We begin each weekly session with one of these relaxation techniques followed by a

Stress Response Awareness

We attempt to raise participants' awareness of various aspects of the stress response process, including the following:

- frequently occurring stressors
- common signs of stress responses (in affective, cognitive, behavioral, somatic, and interpersonal domains)
- how tension manifests in the body
- the thought processes (cognitive appraisals) that precede stress responses and the ways in which they distort stressful stimuli
- the coping responses used most frequently in stressful situations
- characteristic ways of dealing with negative emotions such as anger
- nuances of interpersonal styles of conflict resolution
- social support resources

script featuring relaxing imagery (e.g., a tropical beach, a rain forest scene) designed to deepen the relaxation experience. At the end of the session, participants are given a homework assignment using either written instructions or an audiotape that takes them through one of the relaxation techniques that they have just learned. We strongly recommend that this tape be created using one of the group leaders' voices because our patients have stated that they strongly prefer this method.

AIM 3: MODIFYING COGNITIVE APPRAISALS

Our third aim is to teach participants ways to modify their appraisals of stressful events. This skill is a critical building block for using the other cognitive, behavioral, and interpersonal techniques introduced later in the program. Primarily, we use cognitive therapy techniques such as cognitive restructuring and rational thought replacement (Beck, Rush, Shaw, & Emery, 1979). Weekly sessions include didactic material, in-session exercises (awareness raising exercises, role-plays), and homework assignments designed to increase participants' awareness of the links between thoughts and emotions and physical changes, enhance their familiarity with their distorted appraisals of stressful events, and teach them how to replace identified cognitive distortions with rational interpretations of stressful events. The homework assignments ask participants to list the most stressful events that occurred during the week and their cognitive appraisals and emotional responses to those events. As they progress through the weekly sessions, participants continue to monitor their cognitive appraisals, rational thought replacements, and subsequent emotional responses to weekly events as they occur.

AIM 4: BUILDING COPING SKILLS AND INCREASING EMOTIONAL EXPRESSION

Our fourth aim is to help participants challenge and change the cognitive, behavioral, and interpersonal coping strategies that they have been using to deal with stressful events and conflicting relationships. We first attempt to raise participants' awareness of inefficient ways that they may have developed for coping with stressors and the ways they express their feelings in response to stressful situations. In addition to raising awareness levels, we use a coping skills training strategy to show group members ways to challenge old coping responses. During a period of several weeks, participants learn to replace less efficient, indirect coping strategies with various direct, emotion- and problem-focused coping strategies. They also learn about the situations in which different forms of direct strategies are likely to be most effective (Folkman et al., 1991). They are offered didactic lessons about stress and coping theory and in-session exercises designed to broaden their awareness of available coping options. In homework assignments, they are given the opportunity to identify and label the less efficient coping strategies that they used in response to stressors encountered that week. They are then instructed to generate alternative coping responses that may have been more efficient in minimizing the magnitude and duration of the resulting stress response.

Once participants are sufficiently aware of the ways in which they typically cope with stressors and some of the available alternatives, they participate in sessions specifically focused on handling and communicating negative emotions such as anger and ways to resolve interpersonal conflict. Participants first engage in exercises designed to increase their awareness of the sorts of stressors and situations that get them most angry and the ways that they are able to detect angry feelings. We also attempt to increase participants' awareness of the ways in which they characteristically express their anger toward others and the likely consequences of this expression. In-session exercises are used to raise participants' awareness of their patterns of angry responses, the role of situational factors in decisions to express anger, and the role of internal factors (e.g., hunger, sleep loss) in the anger experience, and the various components of the anger appraisal process. The group generates alternative anger responses and then learns how to modify their responses.

Another session addressing Aim 4 attempts to broaden the stress management techniques used for anger to the general area of conflict resolution. Participants are provided with didactic material and exercises designed to increase their awareness of several different communication styles and the likely consequences of using them in various conflicting interpersonal situations. The group then engages in a discussion about the advantages and disadvantages of each of these styles. During in-session role-playing, the participants use various conflict resolution styles (e.g., aggressive, passive, passive–aggressive, assertive) while reading scripted interpersonal exchanges with other group members. Role-playing helps participants become more aware of the emotional sequelae of using the various forms of communication. In the remainder of this session, we discuss some common reasons for using unassertive behaviors and then review how to send more assertive messages. The homework assignment asks participants to record at least three problem situations that occurred during the week and were related to communication (e.g., sharing with partner, discussing treatment options with health care providers, arguing with family members). They are then asked to list their cognitive appraisals of and immediate emotional responses (and their intensity) to the situations. They then list their behavioral responses and classify them (as assertive, aggressive, passive, or passive–aggressive). Finally the participants are asked to insert an alternative assertive response when needed and evaluate how it might have changed their emotional response and accompanying cognitive appraisals. In so doing, participants are able to practice identifying elements of their personal style that they may want to change. They also get the opportunity to integrate the skills learned in this session with the other CBSM techniques that they have learned in prior sessions. One key goal that we seek to achieve is increasing patients' awareness of the connections that exist among cognitive, behavioral, and interpersonal stress response processes.

AIM 5: REDUCING SOCIAL ISOLATION

Having provided participants with opportunities to increase their awareness of their stress response processes and multiple aspects of stressors, modify their cognitive appraisals of stressors, and build cognitive, behavioral, and interpersonal coping skills, the final aim focuses on ways to reduce social isolation by identifying and using beneficial sources of social support. We present a social support session in the 7th week of the program. It begins by defining social support and discussing the difference sources of social support that people encounter. Participants complete a self-study of social support, and the group proceeds to discuss participants' relative satisfaction with their support in the areas of emotional support, financial support, and guidance. They also discuss examples of the ways in which they provide support for other people.

Group leaders then present didactic information on several of the ways in which supportive relationships might enhance quality of life and possibly benefit health. Direct benefits discussed include the areas of informational support and tangible (e.g., financial) support, whereas indirect benefits discussed include the stress-buffering role of emotional support. Participants then work together to generate a list of potential obstacles to maintaining a strong support network and determine to what extent they have personal control over these obstacles. We then attempt to integrate CBSM techniques with the social support topic by asking participants to challenge (and possibly reframe) their cognitive appraisals about their decisions to use or avoid a specific social support source, modify (as appropriate) their coping strategies for seeking out and using support, and then reevaluate how these changes might alter their emotional state and quality of life.

The program ends with a short review of the five aims of the B-SMART program (increasing awareness, reducing anxiety and tension, modifying cognitive appraisals, building coping skills and expressing emotions, and reducing social isolation) and the various CBSM techniques used to achieve those goals (e.g., body scans, relaxation and imagery techniques, cognitive restructuring, coping skills, anger management and assertiveness techniques, social network building). Participants then complete a personal plan for implementation and maintenance of the techniques they have learned and receive a month's supply of self-monitoring materials that they will turn in at regular 6-month follow-ups.

WHY USE A GROUP FORMAT?

We developed the B-SMART program as a closed, structured intervention group of six to eight people. The group meetings last for 2 hours and are held once weekly for 10 weeks, with the group being facilitated by two group leaders. The first portion of each session focuses on relaxation and imagery skills, and the second portion focuses on a set of CBSM techniques. Each session begins and ends with a review of a homework assignment. To maximize the effectiveness of this intervention with the target population, we allow participants to generate examples of recent psychosocial stressors to be used during in-session behavioral role playing. We also encourage all group members to practice newly learned relaxation techniques at home on a daily basis and record the frequency and effectiveness of these experiences on self-monitoring cards.

The B-SMART program is designed to be implemented by two group leaders who are experienced in conducting group psychotherapy and have been trained in the specifics of the program using the accompanying *Therapist's Manual* and directed readings. The program uses group leaders and group members as coping role models, which facilitates positive social comparisons and demonstrates a real-life use of social support for informational purposes. It is our hope that people responding particularly well to this aspect of the program might leave a session with thoughts such as, "I saw *her* do it, so I can too," "I'm glad to hear that someone else has these crazy thoughts," or "It's good to know that I can rely on these people for some honest feedback and guidance." The supportive group environment used in our program also encourages the honest expression of feelings and provides a regular opportunity for participants to obtain emotional support. Although the responses discussed deal mainly with the informational aspects the group interaction process, the emotional aspects we emphasize involve nurturance, unconditional positive regard, reassurance of worth, and a general sense that group members can rely on each other at any time. Emotional support is more fluid and potent in groups that are cohesive and communal (Yalom & Greaves, 1977). We have reasoned that group interventions directed toward people attempting to manage the same chronic problem or disease enhance the built-in sense of community that allows group members to express their feelings more freely.

Within the group context, we also hope that the program can replace feelings of powerlessness and isolation with a sense of mastery and altruism. Attempting to achieve personal mastery and observing others in the group master their own obstacles can bolster self-efficacy, which may help participants in other situations. Although our program's instructions to the participants about how to change their thinking and behaviors are an important and useful blueprint, it is their own belief in their ability to overcome adversity that allows them to dig the first hole, pour the cement for the foundation, and execute the building plan. We hope that giving participants the opportunity to witness testimonials and personally experience the effects that other group members have had after changing the way they view stressors will set this process in motion. It is also well known that such group interventions are often successful because they provide people with the opportunity to become altruistically involved in the lives of others. Knowing that discussing their old, ineffective strategies and discovering new ones are helping their fellow group members, people in the B-SMART program may feel less defensive about disclosing personal or potentially embarrassing information and may finish the group sessions with a renewed sense of self-worth and belonging.

The final mission of the group is to discourage avoidance and denial of current problems and to encourage more direct actions such as cognitive restructuring, active problem solving, doing relaxation exercises, and seeking social support. The program provides didactic material and awareness exercises in each session and also relies on feedback from group members to achieve this goal. A salient feature of this program is that it encourages group members to monitor ongoing stressful events and use examples of them for in-session exercises that involve all group members. For instance, after group members recognize and record an incident involving a cognitive distortion or unassertive behavioral response, they are encouraged to act out the situation with another group member while the other members provide feedback observations. This step increases members' awareness of the subtleties of different coping responses.

In summary, the group format allows members to use and benefit from certain processes that would not be available in individual psychotherapy. Most importantly, they are able to use group members and group leaders as coping role models and for positive social comparisons, they can observe the use of social support for informational purposes, they are in an atmosphere that encourages emotional expression, and they have the opportunity to seek emotional and instrumental social support from the other group members in a semipublic yet safe and confidential environment. The true efficiency of the group format can be maximized for the purpose of modeling as well as teaching all of the previously noted components that constitute the aims of the B-SMART program.

OTHER FORMAT CONSIDERATIONS

Stress Response Efficiency

Implicit in all of the treatment sessions is the importance of increasing awareness of the automatic yet controllable responses to stressors and burdens. We tell participants that by the end of the program, we would like them to become experts at understanding their own stress responses. In so doing, we emphasize the notion that they can continue to improve their skill and efficiency at managing the inevitable collection of stressors that will develop on a daily basis as they deal with having breast cancer. As mentioned previously, it is very difficult to adopt a new, untested coping strategy without first stepping back and becoming more aware of the failure of our old strategies to resolve burdens, the sense of helplessness resulting from their circular path, and the repeated results of their destructive consequences The didactic segments and written handouts accompanying most of the weekly sessions are designed to catalyze this awareness process. However, we have observed that some of the most potent ways that people become more aware of these subtle processes is by doing homework assignments in which they track their own thoughts and feelings accompanying stressful encounters, report them back to the group, listen to other group members discuss their own distortions during the group sessions, and watch the members think of and model more appropriate coping responses.

Coping Options

When developing this intervention, we attempted to minimize the degree to which it seemed to be "preachy" or dogmatic to the participants. This is important because treatment adherence is likely to be better if participants sense that they have choices when they are dealing with stressful situations. Another reason for leaving participants some freedom in their choice of different stress management techniques is that dogmatic recommendations for stress management and lifestyle changes may cause participants to feel guilty if their initial efforts at modifying their responses to stressors are unsuccessful (e.g., they still feel somewhat anxious). One subtlety of the B-SMART program is that it includes a combination of problem-focused (e.g., assertiveness, active coping) and emotion-focused (e.g., relaxation training, seeking emotional support) coping options. We deemed this aspect to be important for several reasons. First, it is well known that people use a blend of coping strategies; neither emotion- nor problem-focused strategies are the sole answer to all situations. Thus, we hoped to enhance the program's usefulness in real-world situations by weaving both types of responses into the program. Second, people differ (based on their core personality style) in their preferred set of coping strategies. For example, some are not entirely comfortable with emotion-focused strategies. Interventions that fail to offer the opportunity to match personality style with coping strategy may be ineffective. We regularly encourage people to use the CBSM techniques that are most helpful to them. Third, people are likely to differ in the degree to which they think they have personal control over current life demands. Emotion-focused strategies are believed to be most effective for uncontrollable situations, and problem-focused strategies are the most effective for controllable situations (Folkman et al., 1991). By providing people with a blend of each type of strategy, our hope is that this program will improve individuals' ability and "flex-ability" to deal with the wide range of changeable or controllable versus unchangeable or uncontrollable burdens that are a necessary part of living with breast cancer and its treatment.

In addition to using these techniques, we have also found it helpful to weave certain topics and pieces of information into the group sessions to stimulate the use of the CBSM skills such as cognitive restructuring. In the past, the topics that have been most effective have included learning about the behavioral and medical aspects of dealing with breast cancer, negotiating responsibilities with family members, and discussing job-related stressors. The specific topic areas chosen for use in a given group depend to some degree on the life situation of the majority of the participants. For instance, in groups primarily made up of employed individuals, job stress may be a key catalyst for many group discussions and applications. However, members of groups in which the majority is unemployed may respond better to discussions about financial burdens, family issues, and personal relationships as salient sources of stress.

Intervention Content

As noted previously, the B-SMART program is made up of a 10-part series of weekly sessions that are designed to address five therapeutic aims. We have packaged each session into two segments: (a) a 45-minute relaxation portion at the beginning of the session and (b) a 90-minute stress management portion (includes a 15-minute break). The following section describes the rationale for the relaxation and stress management strategies and specific techniques that are introduced during the 10 weekly sessions of the program.

RELAXATION STRATEGIES

Relaxation Techniques and Anxiety Reduction

As described in preceding sections, stress responses are often characterized by sympathetic nervous system (SNS) activation and concomitant activity in the sympathetic adrenomedullary (SAM) and hypothalamic–pituitary–adrenocortical (HPAC) systems. Affective processes such as anxiety often accompany these responses and may manifest themselves in physical symptoms. Progressive muscle relaxation was originally developed by Jacobson (1938) as a means of counteracting muscle tension symptoms of anxiety.

Relaxation Techniques and Physiological Stress Indicators

Much of the empirical evidence for the influence of relaxation training on SNS-related indexes comes from studies of patients with hypertension. Several investigators have reported decreases in their blood pressure (relative to control patients) when using relaxation training with biofeedback (McGrady et al., 1987; Patel & North, 1975), relaxation with and without biofeedback (Goldstein, Shapiro, & Thananopavarn, 1984), and relaxing imagery with and without cognitive stress management techniques (Crowther, 1983). In addition to blood pressure effects, McGrady et al. (1987) also reported that relaxation training was associated with significant decreases in urinary and plasma cortisol levels among people with hypertension. It is noteworthy that the beneficial effects of relaxation training on hypertension have been demonstrated to be independent of expectancy effects (C. B. Taylor, Farquhar, Nelson, & Agras, 1977).

Progressive muscle relaxation training combined with biofeedback also significantly improved glucose tolerance in a group of people with

Relaxation Strategy Studies

Techniques designed to bring about states of psychological and physical relaxation have been examined for their effectiveness in treating various physical problems including headache (Andrasik, Blanchard, Neff, & Rodichok, 1984; Brown, 1984), hypertension (Crowther, 1983; McGrady et al., 1987; Patel, Marmot, & Terry, 1981), peptic ulcer disease (Aleo & Nicassio, 1978; Brooks & Richardson, 1980), and Raynaud's disease (Jacobson, Manschreck, & Silverberg, 1979; Surwit et al., 1978). The impetus for such investigations has been the increasing evidence that psychosocial factors such as stress can influence the physiological mechanisms controlling some of the symptoms related to these conditions.

non-insulin-dependent diabetes relative to a no-treatment control group (Surwit & Feinglos, 1983). Neither insulin secretion nor action changed as a result of treatment, so it is likely that hepatic glucose uptake increased, suggesting that relaxation training effects may have been mediated by decreased SNS activity. Direct evidence for the effects of relaxation on specific SNS-related indexes is provided by several studies. Among healthy individuals, PMR produced greater reductions in galvanic skin responses than listening to neutral material (Brandt, 1973). In other work, PMR resulted in greater decreases in heart rate, respiration, and electromyographic (EMG) activity than self-relaxation and was able to reduce heart rate and EMG activity more than hypnotic relaxation (Paul, 1969). However, other studies found no differences in the effects of PMR and music on blood pressure (R. I. Edelman, 1970) or in the effects of PMR and nonspecific discussion on blood flow, EMG, and heart rate (Mathews & Gelder, 1969). In a review of the physiological effects of PMR, Borkovec and Sides (1979) concluded that this is the most effective method for inducing autonomic nervous system (ANS) changes when the program involves several sessions and is subject controlled and when physiological overactivity is a pathognomic aspect of a presenting problem. The B-SMART program incorporates several different relaxation-based techniques in addition to PMR in the 10-week program. The major relaxation components of the program are listed in the following display.

PMR

In the first 45-minute segment of the initial four weekly sessions, members receive training in PMR using the program developed by Bernstein

Relaxation Components of the B-SMART Program

- PMR: PMR involves systematically tensing and relaxing the various muscle groups of the body.
- Deep Breathing: Participants learn slow, diaphragmatic (abdominal) breathing, which is contrasted with fast, shallow, chest breathing—breathing that may exacerbate anxiety.
- Guided Visualization: Leaders guide participants through a relaxing beach scene. Later, participants are encouraged to develop their own relaxing scene images.
- Autogenic Training: Autogenics incorporates suggestions of warmth and heaviness and combines them with relaxing suggestions, such as, "My heartbeat is calm and regular."

and Borkovec (1973). This portion of the program starts by training participants to relax by tensing and releasing each of seven muscle groups in the first session and gradually reduces the muscle groups to four. Patients are finally taught to relax their entire body through a countdown procedure. This progressive aspect enables people to monitor their improving ability to control tension levels during the 10-week program. Because this approach culminates in a relatively simple, quick, and easy-to-engage counting cue for relaxation, people may be more likely to continue using it after the program has ended. We recommend that group members practice these exercises twice daily, preferably in the same location (e.g., in a quiet place during their lunch break and at home in the evening). We also ask that they (a) record how often they practice the relaxation exercise and (b) use a subjective 7-point scale to indicate how much tension, or stress, they were feeling immediately before and after their relaxation exercise. This information is recorded on cards or sheets, which are turned in at the beginning of each relaxation session.

Guided Imagery

After group members have completed several weeks of relaxation training, they learn about an imagery component involving a beach scene to enhance the depth of their relaxation experience. They are given an audiotape featuring one of the group leaders reciting an imagery script describing a peaceful beach scene. They are asked to listen to the tape (preferably with headphones) after completing their daily PMR exercises. In addition to the beach scene imagery, we guide participants through several other scenarios including various other nature-related themes (e.g., a rain forest scene). This step can be facilitated by providing participants with an audiotape containing these additional guided imagery passages. We have reasoned that furnishing participants with these imagery audiotapes makes the daily relaxation exercises more interesting and may promote more focused relaxation because auditory distractions are less likely (when headphones are used). It is also plausible that listening to the group leader's voice (which group members have previously associated with relaxation) may result in a conditioned response—one that might be particularly helpful for participants who continue to use these tapes after the groups have ended.

Other Relaxation Techniques

In addition to PMR and imagery, we use several other techniques designed to reduce tension, including autogenic training, deep breathing techniques, and various forms of meditation. The rationale and steps for implementing each of these techniques are included in the *Therapist's Manual*. By the end of the 10-week program, our goal is to have provided participants enough techniques to allow them to choose the ones that work for them.

STRESS MANAGEMENT STRATEGIES

An important part of each session involves providing information and exercises that teach participants techniques such as cognitive restructuring, coping-skills training, assertion training, anger management, and social support building. Relevant issues such as medications, reactions of children and family members, interactions with health care providers, health insurance issues, job-related stressors, and the nature of stress responses are used as catalysts for discussion and application of newly learned cognitive behavioral techniques. We have paired many of the informational aspects of the program with cognitive–behavioral techniques that are most relevant to the information.

Cognitive-based stress management techniques have been used in numerous ways in the health care field, including in the areas of health promotion and disease prevention, detection, and treatment. Specific applications of cognitive stress management interventions have been developed for chronic illnesses such as asthma (Bartlett, 1983), rheumatoid arthritis (Parker et al., 1987), and peptic ulcer (Brooks & Richardson, 1980). Additionally, cognitive techniques have been targeted at the reduction of postoperative Cesarean-section pain (Baumstark & Beck, 1988), pain associated with cancer (Fishman & Loscalzo, 1987), and control of acute and chronic pain (Weisenberg, 1987). By the mid 1980s, effects of cognitive stress management techniques on general health outcomes had been widely researched, yet few investigations focused on hormonal or immunological changes resulting from the implementation of these strategies. Stressors most consistently associated with immunomodulatory effects in humans included those involving perceived helplessness and loss of control (Baum, McKinnon, & Silvia, 1987; Rodin, 1988) and academic stress (Glaser et al., 1986; Glaser et al., 1987). Additionally, affective changes such as anxiety and depression often accompany these stressors and have also been associated with immune changes (B. Linn, Linn, & Jensen, 1981; M. Stein, Keller, & Schleifer, 1985). Hence, cognitive stress management techniques appear to be reasonable immunomodulatory strategies.

Two basic assumptions underlie the use of CBSM techniques. First, individuals are thought of as active processors rather than passive recipients of stimuli from their environments. When faced with a stressor, individuals ostensibly try to appraise their resources so that they can respond. Therefore, the amount of threat, arousal, or stress people experience is determined by their appraisal of the novel stimuli and perception of available resources (Folkman, 1984; Folkman, Lazarus, Gruen, & DeLongis, 1986; Gall & Evans, 1987; Turk et al., 1986). In addition, cognitions, emotions, behaviors, and the social environment often interact (Beck et al., 1979). Accordingly, cognitions can elicit emotions, decrease tension, cause a behavior, and determine the way the behavior is expressed. Similarly, feelings can facilitate or inhibit the development of cognitions that can affect the behavioral response to the environment as a function of the social context (Turk et al., 1986). The second assumption underlying CBSM is that individuals can be taught new patterns of thinking, feeling, and behaving that will help them achieve a feeling of control over their emotional states and maladaptive behaviors, thereby helping them understand that they are active contributors to their lives, not helpless victims (Turk et al., 1986). According to this perspective, an individual's appraisals, beliefs, attitudes, cognitive coping strategies, and expectancies are important mediators in all realms of health, disease, and responses to treatment (Turk et al., 1986).

The CBSM techniques used in the B-SMART program include cognitive restructuring of maladaptive thoughts, feelings, and behaviors; training in coping skills to improve adaptive coping responses such as active problem solving; and anger management, assertiveness training, and training in other techniques focused on building interpersonal skills. These techniques are designed to change the individual's perceptions of environmental events and their ability to manage the situation. For example, cognitive–behavioral techniques have been used with patients who have cancer pain and whose major sources of distress include uncertain medical status, fear of physical and functional deterioration, pain, and death. In this chronic state of distressing uncertainty—which is not unlike the extended treatment period for breast cancer—patients may need to regain a sense of coherence, meaning, and structure in their lives. Cognitive–behavioral interventions can enhance people's sense of personal control or self-efficacy during various stages of disease adjustment and may thereby meet some of these needs (Fishman & Loscalzo, 1987).

The effects of cognitive therapies on depression and anxiety have also been investigated in several studies. This work is relevant to people dealing with cancer because depression and anxiety seem to be related to people's appraisals of environmental stimuli and immune functioning. B. Linn et al. (1981) found that patients with cancer experiencing stress and anxiety had impaired lymphocyte mitogen responsiveness. Depression has been linked to compromised immunological functioning and the course of some immune-related disease processes. For example, Kemeny, Zegans, and Cohen (1987) found a depressed mood to be associated with decreases in cytotoxic T-cell numbers and increases in the rate of herpes simplex virus (HSV) outbreaks. It is also known that improvements in mood and coping during cognitive–behavioral intervention predict changes in immune function (NKCC) and longer survival in patients with early-stage malignant melanoma who were monitored for 6 years (Fawzy et al., 1993).

Although depression is often referred to as an affective disorder, its symptoms include disturbances in psychological and physiological functioning. Studies have concentrated on two different aspects of depression: (a) changes in cognitions and (b) alterations in neuroendocrine activity. The thoughts of depressed patients have been found to be negatively biased with specific processing errors and excessively rigid idiosyncratic beliefs (Blackburn, Jones, & Lewin, 1986; Kovacs & Beck, 1978). These cognitive distortions are highly correlated with depressed mood, and maintenance of distorted thinking is associated with poor response to treatment among patients who are depressed (A. D. Simons et al., 1984). Conversely, improvements in dysfunctional thinking often accompany recovery from depressive illness, regardless of whether the treatment is pharmacotherapy based or cognitively based. Interestingly, greater cognitive enhancement and less relapse are associated with cognitive interventions (Blackburn & Bishop, 1983; Covi & Lipman, 1987; Murphy, Simons, Wetzel, & Lustman, 1984; Stavynski & Grenberg, 1987). Others have noted that compared with the drug imipramine, cognitive therapy resulted in significantly greater decreases in hopelessness and more improvements in self-concept among nonpsychotic outpatients with depression (Rush et al., 1982). Cognitive-based interventions appear to be effective in reducing the psychological symptomatology associated with depression. Importantly, some of the targets of cognitive therapy, including pessimism, have been associated with lower NKCC in patients at risk for developing cancer (Byrnes et al., 1998).

Dysregulations in neuroendocrine activity have been reported for individuals who are chronically stressed or depressed (Amsterdam,

Maislin, Gold, & Winkour, 1989; Christie et al., 1986; Gold et al., 1986), and failure to suppress cortisol secretion after dexamethasone administration (the dexamethasone suppression test) has been used to diagnose "endogenous" depression (Carroll et al., 1981). Moreover, high cortisol plasma concentrations have been shown to return to normal in patients successfully treated with antidepressants (Carroll, Curtis, & Mendels, 1976) or electroconvulsive therapy (Christie, Whalley, Brown, & Dick, 1982) and cognitive therapy (Christie et al., 1982). These findings, combined with those of Rush et al. (1982), suggest that cognitive-based interventions may alter psychological and physiological functioning among individuals with depression. Despite these impressive findings supporting the efficacy of cognitive therapy among patients with psychiatric conditions, less is known about the psychological and physiological effects of cognitive interventions in groups without psychiatric conditions. However, some evidence suggests that cognitive strategies may alter physical and psychological outcomes among individuals with chronic physical diseases. Two such physical problems—duodenal ulcers (Brooks & Richardson, 1980) and arthritis (Parker et al., 1987)—are believed to be affected by psychosocial stressors and the ameliorative effects of cognitive stress management interventions. It is also now known that CBSM intervention decreases cortisol levels in patients with breast cancer (D. Cruess, Antoni, McGregor, et al., 2000) and men infected with HIV (Antoni, Cruess, Cruess, et al., 2000), and decreases in cortisol levels parallel reductions in depressive symptoms or depressed mood during the intervention.

As noted previously, the five sets of stress management techniques used in the B-SMART program include cognitive restructuring, coping-skills training, assertion training, anger management, and social support building. We spend 1 to 3 weeks training participants how to use each of these techniques. Each new topic is introduced using background information and exercises designed to increase participants' awareness of subtle stress response processes that are addressed by the technique being taught. This step is followed by an introduction to the rationale for the use of the technique and the steps for implementing it. The balance of the session is spent applying the technique to examples of ongoing stressors in the participants' lives. We use role-playing and breakaways into dyads when possible to increase the interactive nature of the experience. The following sections describe the steps for implementing the five sets of techniques in the order in which they are introduced in the B-SMART program.

Cognitive Restructuring

At the heart of nearly all of the CBSM interventions just reviewed is the technique of cognitive restructuring. This technique is used to help participants become aware of, challenge, and ultimately replace self-defeating cognitive appraisals of situations that are hindering their psychological adjustment (Beck & Emery, 1979). Cognitive restructuring is introduced early in the B-SMART program, and like the programs developed by Beck and colleagues (e.g., Beck & Emery, 1979), group members maintain an ongoing daily program in which they monitor stressful events, accompanying emotions, automatic thoughts, and physical and social symptoms of stress. These stress symptoms include their responses to life situations and are categorized in cognitive, emotional, behavioral, social, and physiological domains. The goal is to increase group members' *awareness* of (a) the ways in which they are handling difficult situations and (b) the cues that are the early warning signals.

We encourage people to focus on the link between their thoughts and their feelings. Emotions are largely a result of the way people think about things. For example, before a person can experience an event as upsetting, the person must first process (e.g., filter, magnify, distort) the situation in her or his mind and assign it some personal meaning. If the person's perceptions of the event are exaggerated or distorted in some way, the emotional response may be extreme. Depression and pervasive anxiety can be considered extreme responses in some situations. A handy metaphor for explaining this process to group leaders during training is as follows:

> If music is playing on the radio, and you hear static, the static is not caused by faulty transistors or wiring. Rather, the problem is that you are not accurately tuned to the right frequency. Likewise, you don't have a "screw loose" in your stress processor. Your assessment of the situation is simply off target. Because the radio is intact, correcting the static is a simple matter of making a small tuning adjustment. Because your cognitive faculties remain intact during stressful transactions, you can also make adjustments to your appraisals.

Group leaders may choose to use similar metaphors for explaining the notion of cognitive distortions. When conducting these types of cognitive scans, some important questions we ask participants include "What form do the typical cognitive distortions take? Do certain key words in people's thoughts serve as a clue to their distortions? What do people do once they identify such cues?" Following the work of Beck and colleagues, we introduce participants to some of the more common cognitive distortions. We provide them with a typical academic definition of each distortion and a concrete example of each type of thinking in real-life situations. Some of these distortions (adapted from Burns, 1981) are as follows:

- All-or-nothing thinking (black-and-white thinking): A person who uses all-or-nothing thinking appraises situations in rigid categories; they see no in-between or gray areas. All-or-nothing, or black-and-white, thinking forms the basis of perfectionism. It causes people to fear any mistakes or imperfections because if their performance is less than perfect, they consider themselves total failures; they may feel inadequate and worthless. This type of thinking is unrealistic because life can rarely be explained so definitively. A person using all-or-nothing thinking might say, "You're either for me or against me in my battle against this disease."

- Fortune telling: A fortune teller anticipates that things will turn out badly and feels convinced that the prediction is an already established fact. Fortune telling is like having a crystal ball that foretells only misery. The person imagines that something bad is going to happen even though it may be unrealistic. Someone who is fortune telling would think, "I'm bound to have a recurrence, it's just a matter of time" rather than "I may have a recurrence, but worrying won't change the future. I can make the most of each day and focus on leading a healthy life." A closely related distortion, mind reading, might result in a thought such as, "I'm afraid to tell my brother I have breast cancer because I'm afraid he'll never talk to me again."

- "Should" statements: "Should" and "should not" statements, such as "I should be able to do this all by myself, and I should not ask for help," simply make people feel guilty. "Must" and "ought" statements have the same effect. Directing "should" statements (e.g., "People should know what I need; if they don't, they just don't care about me") toward others leaves the person feeling angry, frustrated, and resentful. Directing them toward oneself creates pressure and additional resentment.

It is important to understand that cognitive distortions come in many forms, tend to occur automatically (without volition), and often precede emotional discomfort. We help individuals become more aware of (a) the situations in which their thinking errors tend to occur, (b) the particular types of thinking errors they have been having (e.g., black-and-white thinking, fortune telling), (c) the connection of the cognitive appraisal with the emotional change, and (d) the ways in which these cognitive–emotional events shaped the resulting behaviors and sense of self-efficacy. Some of the exercises used to build a greater awareness of these interlocking processes are illustrated in the *Therapist's Manual* and *Participant's Workbook*.

After introducing participants to definitions of several common cognitive distortions, we encourage them to contribute their own most commonly encountered distortions and if possible the most recent situation in which they were aware of the distortion and its consequences. After all members appear to have an understanding of the distortions, they begin a continuing weekly assignment in which they record stressful or emotionally uncomfortable events that occur in their daily lives. For each event, we ask them to note the type of emotion that they were experiencing and rate its severity from 1 to 100 on a 100-point scale. They also record the automatic thought that preceded the emotional experience and rate their degree of belief in that thought (0% to 100%). Finally, members are asked to note the physical and social symptoms that accompanied this experience so that they can become more attuned to them and use them as warning signals in future situations. To facilitate their adherence to this exercise, we furnish all group members with Thought Monitoring Sheets similar to those developed by Beck and Emery (1979) and ask them to record at least one automatic thought each day. After members have become adept at identifying these distortions, we teach them ways to constructively alter the thoughts using rational thought replacement. These easy-to-use strategies for replacing dysfunctional cognitive appraisals are adapted from the work of Beck and Emery (1979) and Burns (1981) and are described in detail in the B-SMART *Therapist's Manual*.

Coping-Skills Training

After participants have spent several weeks on the cognitive restructuring aspects of the program, we introduce the concept of coping responses. In the past decade, several theorists have studied how individuals respond, adapt, or cope with demands and difficulties and how these responses can be used to predict their future mental and physical health status. Many have argued that in making such predictions, it is less important to know which types of storms people have endured than it is to know how they endured them. This rationale is buttressed by data supporting the idea that individual differences in coping actions and resources play a substantial role in amplifying, diminishing, or otherwise moderating a wide range of environmental burdens. Moreover, the attraction to studying the coping process is driven by the precision with which coping can be defined and measured, its empirical association with psychosocial and physical changes, its inclusion of a wide range of human experiences, and its role in the dynamic ways in which people interact with their environments (Folkman & Lazarus, 1980).

A comprehensive model of the coping process that was developed by Folkman and Lazarus (1980) was quite instrumental in the development of the coping-skills training portions of the B-SMART program. According to this model, the coping process can be classified into modes and strategies and resources. Modes and strategies include direct and indirect strategies, which vary in the degree to which they focus on the source of a problem (problem-focused coping) or on the feelings evoked by the problem (emotion-focused coping). While it is not our intent to exhaust all the possible combinations of these categories, some of the modes and strategies are common to several extant stress management packages, including our B-SMART program.

Direct coping strategies that are problem focused include problem-solving techniques (i.e., learning how to go from point A to point B in the easiest, least painful way), assertive behaviors (e.g., standing up for one's rights, expressing one's needs, using effective communication skills), and seeking out external sources for information (e.g., approaching other members of one's network of family or friends). As others have pointed out, these strategies affect a person's external environment. On the other hand, other strategies can have a direct impact a person's internal world (i.e., private thoughts). These strategies, which are the focus of stress management packages such as the B-SMART program, include the correcting of thinking errors, or cognitive distortions (Beck & Emery, 1979), and reforming, restructuring, relabeling, or replacing cognitive appraisals of troublesome stimuli.

Another set of coping modes and strategies relevant to stress management are the direct strategies used to remediate feelings evoked by difficult situations. These emotion-focused strategies can be used for tension reduction and include activities such as relaxation exercises and physical (e.g., aerobic training) exercises. Alternatively, verbally expressing anger, sadness, or fears is a direct action that people can use to modulate their emotional reactions. Emotion-focused strategies, including direct strategies for tension reduction and emotional release, are important ingredients of stress management and are incorporated in our CBSM program.

We have generally considered the directed strategies to be useful for buffering the impact of immediate situations (e.g., a woman finding out that she has breast cancer) and longer term situations (e.g., coping with the demands the disease and its treatment). In fact, we designed our CBSM intervention package to teach individuals tangible, direct coping strategies, some of which are problem focused (e.g., problem solving, using assertive behaviors, improving communication skills, and using social support networks) and some of which are emotion focused (e.g., using PMR, using autogenics). In addition to teaching individuals these new skills, we also teach them to become more aware of the environmental conditions and biobehavioral stress signals that should trigger the use of these modes and strategies. By teaching people to become more aware of the situations in which direct coping strategies can be used, stress management interventions such as ours encourage people to become more aware of the less effective modes and strategies they are using to handle their difficulties. These strategies, which are often classified as indirect strategies, can be problem-focused or emotion-focused strategies. Becoming more aware of these automatic reactions and habitual behaviors allows people to replace ineffective strategies with more effective ones.

As just mentioned, indirect strategies can focus on the difficult situation (i.e., be problem focused) and include such strategies as behavioral and cognitive avoidance. As the name implies, behavioral avoidance is rerouting one's life away from an uncomfortable person, place, or activity. This behavior may range from more extreme forms, such as phobias, to the more subtle ways that people find to avoid interpersonal conflicts. Among women with breast cancer, behavioral avoidance may take the form of missing follow-up medical appointments or failing to conduct breast self-exams. Cognitive avoidance involves distraction from or outright denial of the problem at hand and does little to change the nature of the problem. Among women with breast cancer, cognitive avoidance might take the form of failing to spend time thinking about treatment options, which could lead to uninformed, snap decisions about treatment choices.

Other indirect strategies focus on ameliorating the emotional sequelae of environmental burdens and are indirect emotion-focused strategies. These strategies include changes in consumption behaviors, such as increased smoking, eating, and alcohol and recreational drug use. Indeed, these strategies can physically distract a person from the problem at hand. Indirect emotion-focused strategies also include giving up, feeling helpless, or fainting. These strategies are often ineffective for handling problems, and research has shown that they may actually increase depressed feelings and impair bodily systems (e.g., the immune system) that protect people against certain pathogens or help to slow the progression of extant disease processes. For instance, a growing number of studies have found that people with breast cancer who have given up or feel helpless and hopeless have a poorer prognosis and shorter survival (e.g., Watson et al., 1999).

After we have explained some of the different forms of coping strategies to the participants, we conduct an exercise to help them (a) become more aware of the coping responses that they use in stressful circumstances, (b) learn to classify these responses into direct/productive and indirect/nonproductive problem and emotion-focused strategies, and (c) learn how to match specific coping responses with specific stressor (stimulus) appraisals.

We begin by setting up an unlabeled 2 × 2 grid on the display board and ask group members to generate examples of how they handled stressors during the past week (e.g., asked for help, set priorities, got a massage, exercised, watched TV; see Table 3.2). Once the group members

TABLE 3.2

Sample B-SMART Matrix of Coping Options

	Coping options	
	Direct/productive	Indirect/nonproductive
Problem-focused coping	• Ask for help. • Set priorities. • Make lists. • Finish tasks. • Go to work early.	• Skip meals to save time. • Distract self. • Clean house. • Deny that problem exists. • Isolate self.
Emotion-focused coping	• Complain to friends. • Do relaxation exercises. • Take a hot bath. • Get a massage. • Do physical exercise. • Attend a counseling session.	• Stay up late pacing. • Worry and ruminate. • Watch TV. • Go shopping. • Eat. • Drink alcohol or take drugs.

have generated several examples, we list them in their correct position in the matrix and add the following labels to the two columns: left column—direct/productive; right column—indirect.nonproductive. We explain that we can classify some coping options as productive (designed to deal directly with some aspect of a stressful experience) or nonproductive (usually designed to avoid dealing directly with the stressor). In addition to labeling the columns, we label the two rows: top row—problem focused; bottom row—emotion focused. We explain that the problem-focused row includes strategies designed to change the problem that is causing the stress, whereas the strategies listed in the emotion-focused row are involved in regulating (e.g., reducing, soothing) their emotional response to the stressful situation. Once the labels have been added, we review the information in each of the four cells. Some typical participant responses are included in Table 3.2.

We explain to the participants that all of the entries in the matrix are individual coping responses. After the group members have had time to become comfortable using the matrix of coping options to categorize their personal response choices, the next step is to introduce the idea that their appraisals of stressors (stimulus) are affected by the controllable and uncontrollable aspects of the stressors. Participants then consider the controllable and uncontrollable aspects of their stressors and how they affected their appraisals. The participants should list the aspects (stressor aspects) on the board next to the response matrix. We then explain to participants that controllable aspects of stressors are best handled with direct/productive problem-focused coping strategies, whereas the uncontrollable aspects are best handled with direct/productive emotion-focused coping strategies. The participants first identify some of the controllable and uncontrollable aspects of a recent stressful experience and the coping responses that they used to dealing with it. We then help them match some controllable aspects of recent stressors with appropriate productive problem-focused coping strategies. We also help them match some uncontrollable aspects of recent stressors with appropriate productive emotion-focused coping strategies.

We end the coping-skills training sessions by explaining that unfortunately, indirect coping strategies are often connected and perpetuate one another. That is, the use of indirect problem-focused strategies often results in the use of indirect emotion-focused strategies and vice versa. In other words, indirect coping responses often run in a closed loop or in a vicious reinforcing cycle. Increases at one end or the other of the cycle are the rule rather than the exception because habitual coping often makes people feel safe, therefore and may actually be driven by the activities that precede and follow them. This process can lead people to become stuck, as they continue to use less adaptive indirect coping strategies such as consuming too much alcohol. Simply telling people to break their bad habits, stand up to their fears, or clean up their act may do little more than remind them of how helpless they are to change things.

Interestingly, other detrimental processes may be initiated by the vicious reinforcing cycle of indirect modes and strategies. Feelings of low self-efficacy that are caused by the cycle of events may affect other areas of people's lives, possibly triggering cognitive distortions (e.g., "I'll always be second-rate"), unassertive responses (e.g., "I have no right to expect more"), and social isolation (e.g., "I don't need any help from anyone"). These cognitive spin-offs from the vicious cycle of indirect coping strategies are targets of stress management programs such as ours. We try to help individuals become more aware of their use of indirect strategies, understand that the strategies do little to control their environments but much to hinder them, and understand that the costs of using the strategies outweigh the benefits. This awareness helps many people become more willing to consider more adaptive strategies. The overarching goal of the coping-skills training sessions is for participants to develop controllability-matched direct/productive problem- and emotion-focused coping strategies to replace habitual and less effective indirect strategies.

Anger Management

Because of the multitude of problems that result from having breast cancer and because of the inappropriate reactions of friends and family members to the diagnosis, patients with breast cancer often experience various difficult emotions including anger, fear, sadness, and anxiety. Some women are very angry and frustrated about having breast cancer because they have always maintained a healthy lifestyle. Other women are infuriated by the lack of understanding from their husbands or family members when they attempt to minimize feelings of loss and fear. Because these emotional experiences (and their sources) can seem so pervasive and overwhelming, people with cancer may feel unable to express their feelings freely, so they end up internalizing, or "stuffing," their anger and frustration. On the other hand, some people may feel so overwhelmed that they express their feelings inappropriately and indiscriminately, making it difficult to be around them. One important aspect of the B-SMART stress management intervention is that it gives women the opportunity to express their frustrations, grief, fears, and other painful emotions, which in turn may facilitate the development of cognitive insights and resolution of distress (Antoni et al., 2001). In addition to helping people process stressful events and losses, some evidence shows that expressing negative emotions in a supportive environment may influence some aspects of immune system functioning (Esterling, Antoni, Fletcher, Margulies, & Schneiderman, 1994; Esterling, Antoni, Kumar, & Schneiderman,1990; Lutgendorf, Antoni, Schneiderman, & Fletcher, 1994; Pennebaker et al., 1988).

People who do not freely express negative or painful emotions may be using some type of avoidance strategy. Our research indicates that avoiding stressful stimuli has deleterious effects on mood (increased anxiety and depression) and immune system functioning in healthy individuals (Lutgendorf et al., 1994) and men who have just been told that they are infected with HIV (Lutgendorf et al., 1997). In addition to the association between use of avoidance strategies and short-term changes in immunological status, we also found increased use of denial coping affects immune status. Men who used denial after being informed that they were infected with HIV had greater impairments in their immunological status at the 1-year follow-up and a greater likelihood of AIDS or death at the 2-year follow-up (Ironson et al., 1994). Dysregulation theory predicts that selective inattention to, avoidance of, or denial of bodily sensations such as pain and emotional states such as distress disrupts the normal negative feedback properties of these phenomena, resulting in up-regulation of distress signal strength by bodily systems. This up-regulation can increase a person's physiological reactivity to and protract recovery from stressors (Jamner & Schwartz, 1986). It may be that avoidance strategies and denial of bodily sensations produce more dysregulation than the initial stressor itself. This suggests that stress management strategies that help people express their feelings may be beneficial for people with breast cancer and other life-threatening diseases. Therefore, two sessions in the B-SMART program—anger management and assertiveness training—use cognitive-based techniques to teach participants how to express negative feelings in the context of their interpersonal relationships.

We have found that anger and frustration are among the most common difficult emotions experienced by women with breast cancer in the B-SMART program. The point of the anger management session is not to challenge the validity of women's perceptions of the sources of their angry feelings; in most cases the participants are correct in their interpretations. Rather, the anger management session focuses on building skills to handle the feelings. These skills focus on increasing awareness of sources of anger and the ways in which each person's angry responses take form, teaching participants ways to slow down the automatic anger reaction and conduct an anger appraisal, and exploring the many options available for expressing anger.

As part of the in-session exercises, participants complete a self-evaluation questionnaire designed to increase their awareness of the sources of anger in their lives and their characteristic anger expression patterns. This exercise and the ensuing discussion give group members the opportunity to discover their "anger buttons," explore their feelings about the ways they express their anger and react to others' anger, and discuss which aspects of their anger management they would like to change. We also discuss ways in which participants can use physical cues (e.g., increased heart rate, muscle tension) as signals of anger. We also discuss the importance of power dynamics in an angry exchange (e.g., arguing with a spouse vs. arguing with a supervisor) and the role of other factors, such being tired, all of which can affect how a person chooses to express feelings.

Participants learn a step-by-step strategy for expressing their angry feelings constructively and are provided with a long list of alternative responses to use in anger-inducing situations. The session ends with a homework assignment in which participants are asked to list a new situation or the most common (repeating) situations that arouse anger in them. They are also asked to list their characteristic physical responses to these situations (physical cues), their characteristic self-talk (for anger appraisals), and an alternative response that they could use instead of the angry response (e.g., cooling down for a few moments, asking for more information).

Assertiveness Training

Assertiveness training is introduced in the session immediately after the session on anger management. We include assertion training in our B-SMART program for the same reason we include anger management. If people cannot communicate their emotions and behavioral intentions to others (including coworkers, family members, friends, and romantic partners), then interpersonal conflict is likely and will continue to persist. Because such conflict can create acute problems (e.g., hostile reactions) or chronic problems (e.g., resentment), emotional, physical, and social symptoms of stress responses may develop. Responding assertively to such situations may substantially decrease these conflicts and their accompanying "stress" symptoms.

To raise participants' awareness of assertiveness, we introduce group members to four styles of communication: unassertive (passive), aggressive, passive–aggressive, and assertive. Passive behavior is behavior that allows other people to make a person's choices. Passive behaviors are problematic because they foster dependency and low self-efficacy and often result in hurt feelings, anxiety, and resentment when others make the wrong choices. We also explain that although most people know the difference between being passive and being aggressive, it is very common for people to confuse assertiveness and aggressiveness. It is important to clarify the subtle differences between these two communication styles. We remind group members that aggressive (e.g., hostile) behavior commonly causes others to feel insulted and turned off. Because aggressive behavior denies the rights of others, they feel hurt and offended and are likely to react aggressively or abandon you. Aggressive exchanges close the channels of communication, hinder negotiations, and often leave both parties feeling tense and isolated—an unpleasant and unhealthy combination.

On the other hand, assertive people exercise their personal rights (e.g., express their feelings) while respecting the rights of others (e.g., listening to their feelings). We emphasize that because assertive exchanges leave the communication channels open, messages are less likely to get lost or distorted, and the communicators remain more relaxed, even during difficult discussions. Because stressful topics are efficiently discussed, resolution may occur more quickly, creating less strain on the relationship and each person.

We also teach people to become more aware of the different emotional, physical, and social sequelae of each form of communication. As in the previous sessions, we stress the importance of using emotional and physical cues of discomfort as an early warning signal that appraisals and coping strategies may need to be changed. Assertiveness training comprises the part of the B-SMART program that teaches people skills for managing interpersonal burdens, difficulties, and challenges.

Building Social Support

Research has shown that social support can moderate the effects of stress on health (Vachon, Lyall, Rogers, Cochrane, & Freeman, 1982; Vachon

Goals of Assertiveness Training

Assertiveness techniques are demonstrated in relation to potential real-life situations such as talking with a physician about a cancer diagnosis and treatment options. The primary goals of this experience are

- to help individuals learn basic communication skills
- to enhance awareness of interpersonal rights
- to encourage expression of opinions and feelings without undue delay, avoidance, or denial

et al., 1980) and physiological indexes (Cobb, 1974; Gore, 1978) including immune functioning (S. Cruess, Antoni, Cruess, et al., 2000). Unemployed men receiving high levels of emotional support from their wives and families have been shown to experience less physiological strain (Gore, 1978) and have lower catecholamine levels (Cobb, 1974) than men with low levels of support. In addition, low social support (e.g., feeling lonely) has been associated with higher urinary cortisol levels, lower NKCC, and lower T-lymphocyte responsiveness (Kiecolt-Glaser et al., 1984). Studies of patients with breast cancer have shown that seeking social support as a major coping strategy and receiving high levels of support from a spouse predict higher NKCC (Levy & Herberman, 1988). Recent findings indicate that improvements in social support during CBSM intervention explain some of its beneficial effects on mood (Lutgendorf et al., 1998) and components of the immune system (S. Cruess, Antoni, Cruess, et al., 2000).

Investigations of hardiness and social support as buffers against illness suggest that the more active components of social support (e.g., engaging and interacting with supportive others), as opposed to passive components (e.g., being distracted from troubles), have the strongest stress-buffering effects (Kobasa, Maddi, Puccetti, & Zola, 1985). Psychosocial interventions that include active engagement in group activities may have the most potent role in stress reduction.

Social support is provided subtly in several aspects of the B-SMART program. The group format may increase perceptions of community and decrease social isolation. Regular participation in role-playing exercises with group members also facilitates cohesiveness among the women. In addition, in Session 7, we focus specifically on raising participants' awareness of resources and limitations in their social networks and strategies for improving specific sources of support.

We have reasoned that once participants learn to handle interpersonal conflict more efficiently through the use of anger management and assertion skills, they might find that they value the frequent exchanges and crave more fulfilling social relationships. Therefore, the social support session of the B-SMART program (which precedes the anger management and assertiveness training sessions) is dedicated to introducing the different types of social support of which group members may be unaware. For example, the session delineates various sources of social support, such as those that provide guidance through difficult times (e.g., instrumental or informational support) and those who regularly offer nurturance and positive regard (i.e., emotional support). Social support is not a single type of assistance. It is a coping resource with many different domains, some of which facilitate certain forms of coping. For instance, financial or physical support might fuel active coping strategies such as problem solving, whereas positive regard or emotional support may help a person to accept, express feelings about, or cognitively reframe a difficult situation.

Group members participate by mapping out the qualitative aspects of their own social support networks. These forms of support may include receiving a loan from a friend, getting useful information, or even just getting cheered up by somebody. After presenting their maps to the group, the members discuss the strengths and weaknesses of various social support channels. We also encourage group-generated strategies for enhancing support systems in subsequent sessions. These strategies are often a synthesis of anger management and assertion techniques. To illustrate how all of the CBSM skills can be integrated to address a specific issue, the following section explains some of the ways that the B-SMART techniques can used to build social support networks.

INTEGRATING DIFFERENT STRATEGIES: BUILDING SOCIAL SUPPORT WITH THE B-SMART PROGRAM

As participants progress through the 10-week program, we encourage them to integrate skills they learned in prior weeks into the new material being covered in each session. Following is a description of one stream of integration that appears to be particularly helpful for participants and can be made explicit in the last group session.

Increasing Awareness of Social Network Qualities

The first step involves increasing the participants' awareness of their support network *strengths and weaknesses* and the importance of social support. First, we discuss how socially connected participants are to their family, friends, and community. We then determine the availability of the support and how helpful the support is when it is received. We also assess how proactive the participants are in getting support when they need it and how successfully they communicate their needs to members of the social network. Objective assessment devices such as the Social Provisions Scale (Russell, Cutrona, Rose, & Yurko, 1984) may be useful for clarifying the areas from which participants regularly receive social support and the areas from which they do not. A final step in the assessment process involves determining which factors could prevent group members from obtaining or maintaining a strong support network. Once these obstacles have been clearly delineated, we ask the individuals to rate the controllability, or changeability, of each of these stressors. The stressors that can be modified can be addressed using various intervention strategies learned in prior sessions of the program. We also discuss with participants strategies (emotion focused) for dealing with uncontrollable obstacles so that these barriers will not have an unnecessarily powerful and detrimental influence on their lives.

Challenging Cognitive Appraisals

After increasing participants' awareness of their support network strengths and weaknesses, the group leaders can then use interventions that will address difficulties accessing the network. In one powerful intervention, which is modeled after Beck and Emery's (1979) model of cognitive therapy, the group leader challenges participants' cognitive appraisals about why it is difficult to form social connections with supportive others. This intervention usually begins with the group leaders asking participants to think of people in their social network with whom they have not shared concerns or who they have not approached for help since their diagnosis. The participants who are able to identify such people can review the obstacles involved in those relationships. This intervention involves a technique of eliciting the automatic negative thoughts and cognitive distortions that convince the participants they are undeserving of or unable to form social bonds with these people. Only then can the group leaders help the participants reframe their thoughts more rationally so that they can be more realistic and proactive in establishing and maintaining social relationships.

Some rational thought replacements might include

- "Maybe my family won't be as harsh and critical as I am expecting them to be."
- "Perhaps my family won't fall apart if they become aware of how vulnerable I am feeling."
- "Although seeing other people sick with cancer can be scary for family members, helping me out with things can actually make them feel more useful and less helpless."

▪ "I know that I sometimes withdraw from people when I am under stress. Has this been a useful behavior for me in the past? Has this made me feel better?"

As participants discover and challenge these insidious cognitive distortions, the group leaders can help them change the various negative thought patterns in their effort to enhance self-esteem and become an advocate for their own social support.

Teaching Interpersonal Coping Strategies

Another useful intervention involves educating participants about the various coping strategies that they can use to improve and enhance their support network. Of course, the potential usefulness of these strategies may depend to some degree on the personality and cultural characteristics of participants and the stressful nature of their circumstances. Relevant sessions from the B-SMART program include those focusing on identifying problem-focused and emotion-focused coping strategies, learning effective methods for expressing negative emotions such as anger, and learning assertive communication techniques. Each of these sets of skills can have a substantial effect on the level of benefits participants receive from members of their social network. For instance, group leaders teach assertiveness skills to enable participants to seek out information, obtain tangible aid (e.g., money, instructions, advice), and communicate needs and feelings (good and bad) more clearly to friends, family, and supportive others (e.g., medical personnel).

We also encourage participants to accept needed help from members of their support network. (This is often difficult for people who have always considered themselves to be independent.) They can also be encouraged to rely on trusted friends and family members for comfort, love, nurturance, and companionship (Spiegel, 1993) to enhance self-esteem and feelings of social connection. Participants are also encouraged to find people with whom they can discuss uncensored thoughts and feelings openly (Spiegel, 1993). This step can be accomplished by (a) relying on existing relationships with others, (b) rekindling dormant relationships, and (c) relying on religious organizations or support agencies.

Some participants may have less difficulty finding people to serve as social supports but more difficulty effectively communicating their emotional needs to them. Several activities in the B-SMART program are designed to help participants become more aware of their emotional state and more accurately identify the fears and frustrations that underlie the feelings. After they increase their awareness, they need to develop the tools to communicate their emotional needs. Using interpersonal skills such as assertiveness and anger management that they have learned in the B-SMART program may help them communicate their emotional needs. Recent evidence also suggests that writing down thoughts and feelings about traumatic or stressful events may enhance immune function (Antoni, 1997; Esterling et al., 1990, 1994; Lutgendorf et al., 1994; Pennebaker et al., 1988). Thus, participants who would like to keep a journal are encouraged to do so. In addition, sharing their journal with another person could improve the level of intimacy in an existing relationship. Finally, the act of writing may be associated with immunological changes that could possibly improve their health status during and after adjuvant therapy.

Research has also shown that pets, which can be important sources of companionship, may exert a powerfully relaxing effect on the body (e.g., by lowering blood pressure), thus producing possible psychological and physical health benefits. Participants who enjoy being around animals are encouraged to adopt a pet. If they already have one, they can simply be reminded of the wonderful source of support and companionship that they have.

Accessing Resources

Participants are also encouraged to increase their involvement in the community (e.g., by becoming involved in cancer-related groups) so that they will feel helpful. Feeling that they are able to give back the support they have received (which is not possible with medical personnel) can empower them and increase their self-esteem (Hays, Chauncey, & Tobey, 1990). Teaching the participants more effective ways to communicate could also help them give their family members more productive ways to provide emotional and instrumental support. The participants could also learn how to encourage family members to be physically present and available whenever possible (Dakof & Taylor, 1990).

Because of the importance of peers in the support networks of patients with cancer, participants are encouraged to approach community organizations that promote the involvement of people who have previously had cancer (e.g., as peer helpers, as sources of support for people who lack supportive peer networks). This can also help prevent burnout among participants who are currently functioning as caregivers. Programs that use support providers (e.g., drop-in centers, buddy programs, telephone hotlines) or bring people together in a supportive context (e.g., mutual support groups) can be valuable methods for facilitating peer relationships. As part of the B-SMART program, we provide group members with information on several formal support organizations in the community. However, we are aware that some patients do not want to identify themselves as "cancer survivors" and are attracted to the B-SMART program because of its emphasis on stress management skills. For these women, engaging in other types of groups (e.g., groups related to hobbies, sports, or other common interests) may be equally important.

Focusing on Enduring Relationships

One important goal of the B-SMART program is to enhance the social support networks of group participants. An entire session of this program is devoted to understanding and improving social support. In addition, group members learn various other techniques for maintaining and enhancing present relationships, including improving communication skills, changing their perceptions of their interpersonal interactions, learning to deal with intense emotions in relationships (e.g., anger), and changing the ways they cope with the relationship demands. Thus, considerable attention is paid to teaching participants various methods for enriching their existing support networks and bringing more supportive people into their lives.

In addition to the direct benefits of social support enhancement, participation in a group such as the B-SMART program—in which other members have similar medical problems and discuss a topic of common interest—is an indirect source of support. During each session, a considerable amount of time is devoted to group participation and discussion. Group members often report that their strongest bonding experiences occur during these discussions, especially during discussions about anxiety-provoking and frightening situations. They feel encouraged that other people understand and appreciate them and will support them on a weekly basis. The focus on the value of human relationships that develop in a support group sets the stage for the participants' final task—dismantling the group. Each member is given the opportunity to share with the group what they have taken from the 10-week experience and what they plan to do next.

We have chosen to use a finite set of CBSM techniques in the 10-week B-SMART program. Table 3.3 summarizes the sequence of relaxation and stress management components introduced in the B-SMART program during the 10-week intervention. The techniques we have chosen are those that most saliently and directly address the intervention aims of our conceptual model for psychosocial adjustment to breast cancer; we also chose techniques that could be readily used by mental health clinicians who use the accompanying *Therapist's Manual*. It is conceivable that certain professionals may wish to embellish certain aspects of intervention and use exercises with which they are more familiar to achieve

TABLE 3.3

B-SMART Relaxation and Stress Management Components

	Relaxation	Stress Management
Week 1	PMR for 16 muscle groups	Cognitions, stress, and disclosure
Week 2	PMR for seven muscle groups Relaxing imagery	Stress and awareness
Week 3	PMR for four muscle groups Relaxing imagery	Linking thoughts and feelings
Week 4	Passive PMR for four muscle groups Relaxing imagery	Automatic thoughts and cognitive distortions
Week 5	Deep breathing Relaxing imagery	Rational thought replacement
Week 6	Deep breathing Relaxing imagery	Coping skills training
Week 7	Autogenics Relaxing imagery	Social support
Week 8	Autogenics Relaxing imagery	Anger management
Week 9	Meditation Relaxing imagery	Assertion training
Week 10	Participant's choice Relaxing imagery	Summary and review

some of the goals (e.g., use Gestalt techniques to raise awareness). These decisions are best made within the context of specific program goals. We stress that the efficacy of the B-SMART program can be maximized by using a group format, the CBSM techniques reviewed in this text, and weekly meetings, preferably in the proper sequence.

Structure of the Intervention

GROUP MEETINGS AND PROGRAM DURATION

We have designed the B-SMART program to be used in the context of regular (preferably weekly) group meetings supplemented by out-of-session activities such as relaxation practice and various self-monitoring procedures. Although we have held two 60- to 90-minute sessions per week (one relaxation, one stress management), participants prefer to combine the relaxation and stress management sessions into a single 2-

to 2.5-hour session held once weekly. We currently conduct all of our B-SMART groups using this format. Because of the length of these sessions, it is recommended that group leaders begin each session with 45 minutes of relaxation and guided imagery, followed by a 15-minute break, and then the 75-minute stress management portion. Because the program lasts 10 weeks, it is important before the first group meeting to establish a location and meeting time that are convenient for the participants. At this point, participants can discus any prescheduled activities (e.g., adjuvant therapy) that may keep them from attending certain sessions. They are assigned appropriate readings from the *Participant's Workbook* to keep them on schedule.

GROUP SIZE

The optimal size of a B-SMART group is six to eight participants led by two group leaders, a combination that ensures a balance of lively group interactions and monitoring by group leaders. The number of participants can be as few as three without substantially diminishing the effectiveness of group interactions. Groups of larger than eight are not recommended because the size may compromise the group leaders' ability to effectively monitor the program, and group members will not have enough time to participate verbally in each session. Although certain in-session activities do involve small group discussions and role-play dyads, it is not critical to have even-numbered size groups because a group leader can be used to form a dyad in most of the sessions.

CLOSED-GROUP FORMAT

Because the B-SMART program uses a programmed sequence of relaxation-based and stress management techniques that progressively build on one another, it is important that all group members learn the techniques in a specific order. Therefore, the B-SMART sessions should be run using a closed-group format. Although it is occasionally reasonable to allow a participant to join the group meetings in the second weekly session or to miss a meeting later in the program, it is not advisable to run the program as if it were an open-ended, revolving group, with new members joining throughout the 10-week period.

SEQUENCE OF SESSIONS

The types of questions we receive most frequently from group leaders running the B-SMART program are, "How important is it that the program is followed exactly in sequence? Do the techniques have to be introduced in exactly the same order? Can we tailor the program to the individual needs of group members?" Because the program incorporates many different relaxation-based and stress management techniques in the relatively short period of 10 weeks, it is essential that group leaders remain on track during each session and during the 10-session sequence. However, it is also critical that each participant be given the opportunity in each session to apply each newly learned CBSM technique to their own lives. They also need time to review with the group leader any material that they did not fully grasp from prior sessions. We designed the program on the basis of the hypothesis that relaxation-based and stress management techniques can be most effectively introduced in a logical order, progressing from simple, unitary procedures to combinations of different procedures.

SEQUENCE OF RELAXATION TECHNIQUES

We introduce relaxation-based techniques in Session 1 using a very detailed set of instructions for muscle relaxation (PMR). The relaxation exercise uses the major muscle groups and begins with one of the most frequently flexed group of muscles—those controlling the forearm. During this session, participants work through different sets of muscles following the instructions of group leaders. They are asked to practice relaxing these same muscle groups at home during the subsequent week and are given an instruction sheet to help them practice. By the second week, they cluster together certain muscles using a seven-muscle exercise that they can practice at home during the subsequent week. The sequence progresses to a four-muscle exercise by the third week and to a simple counting procedure by the fourth week. All of these procedures are adapted from a longer program developed by Bernstein and Borkovec (1973).

Being reasonably assured that participants have become skilled at relaxing various muscle groups after 4 weeks in the program, we add a guided imagery experience in either the third or fourth week as time permits. During this procedure, the group leader asks participants to imagine a nature scene. They are to try and remain comfortably relaxed with their eyes closed while the group leader talks them through a script depicting the scene (e.g., beach or forest). At this point, participants are given an audiotape with a very similar imagery exercise and are instructed to listen to it (preferably with headphones to minimize extraneous sounds) daily. They are also asked to continue doing the PMR counting procedure or one of the other muscle group relaxation procedures. In subsequent weeks, the group leaders introduce more complex imagery exercises blended with other more powerful techniques such as deep breathing, autogenics, and meditation, and instruct participants to listen to one of the imagery tapes at home. Thus, during the course of the 10-

week program, participants progress from active muscle relaxation to more passive muscle relaxation techniques, to unitary guided imagery experiences combined with relaxation exercises, and finally to imagery procedures combined with deep breathing, autogenics, and meditation.

SEQUENCE OF STRESS MANAGEMENT TECHNIQUES

We teach participants the stress management techniques in a prearranged sequence based on a four-component theory. This model classifies stress management processes into (a) awareness-raising activities, (b) appraisal activities, (c) coping response activities, and (d) coping resource activities. We have reasoned that in addition to learning all of the most effective CBSM techniques available, participants should understand the relationships among these four stress management processes and the ways that they can be used together during stressful interactions. In the first session, we clarify this point by stating that effective stress management involves (a) raising awareness of reactions to stressors, (b) improving the ability to assess stressor appraisals (i.e., thoughts about stressors), (c) making choices about coping or other reactions to stressors, and (d) better utilizing resources to help deal with stressors.

As we try to help participants raise their awareness during the first session, we ask them to identify subtle physical signs of stress that they have experienced personally. After the session, participants are instructed to monitor their stress daily and record their stress levels on wallet-size cards or workbook sheets that they give to their group leader at the next session. During the next session, we build participants' awareness of their stress responses by reviewing common *cognitive* changes (e.g., anxious thoughts, fearful anticipation, poor concentration, memory problems), *emotional* changes (e.g., irritability, restlessness, depression), *behavioral* changes (e.g., avoiding certain tasks; changes in drinking, eating, or smoking patterns), *physical* changes (e.g., stiff or tense muscles, grinding teeth, clenching fists, sweating, tension headaches, difficulty swallowing), and *social* changes (avoiding others, getting easily irritated by others, venting to others) that may occur during a stressful situation. Participants are asked to discuss how they experience changes in these five areas when they are under stress. During this session, participants are also led through various exercises designed to raise their awareness of areas of tension in their body and clarify the connection between changes in emotional states and physical states. During the subsequent week (Session 2), they are asked to monitor various aspects of any stressful situations they experience, including the source of the stress and their associated emotional and physical changes. During the remaining weeks of the program, the theme of "raising awareness" is stressed at the beginning of every session because it is an excellent introduction to techniques such as cognitive restructuring, coping skills training, assertion training, and anger management.

As they address the second major goal of stress management, improving the ability to assess stressor appraisals, participants begin during Session 3 to examine the links between their thoughts and their feelings. The session involves didactic lessons and exercises designed to demonstrate that all emotional experiences (including those associated with stress) are preceded by cognitive activities (appraisals about the stressors). During this session, participants also complete exercises designed to help them more accurately label emotions such as sadness, anger, guilt, and anxiety and the thoughts, or self-talk, that precede these emotions. They also learn that because physical changes often accompany emotional changes, the cognitive appraisals may precede the emotional and physical changes. Subsequent appraisals about their emotional and physical state (e.g., being worried about how tense they feel) can further aggravate the emotional or physical changes, creating a vicious cycle. Finally, the group members learn that one of the most efficient ways to break the positive feedback loop of this vicious cycle is to change their negative, or distorted, appraisals. After the session, participants are asked to complete a written exercise in which they identify their thoughts and feelings in response to several interpersonal scenarios that are included in their *Participant's Workbook*.

In Session 4, participants learn about several of the most common types of cognitive distortions, or negative thoughts (e.g., all-or-none thinking, "should" statements), that people can experience in stressful situations. Using examples of stressors from their own lives, participants are asked to think of some recent occasions when they used one or more of these types of cognitive distortions. During the subsequent week, they complete an at-home exercise in which they identify stressful situations that occurred during the week and, verbatim, the thoughts, emotions, and physical changes that accompanied each situation. They are also asked to categorize each cognitive distortion or negative thought. In the last session dealing specifically with examining cognitive appraisals (Session 5), participants learn the technique of rational thought replacement, which has the following five steps:

- Identify self-talk and cognitive distortions revealed therein.
- Rate your degree of belief in the accuracy of your thoughts.
- Challenge or dispute the self-talk as inaccurate, negative, or otherwise distorted.
- Change the distortion by modifying your self-talk, using a more rational alternative.

▪ Evaluate the outcome according to (a) how much you believe in your new appraisal and (b) any changes in emotional state that you have experienced.

We ask participants to use rational thought replacement to address several stressors that are commonly experienced by women with breast cancer. Participants are asked to use this technique to handle stressors that occur during the subsequent week and to complete monitoring sheets that progress through the five-step rational thought replacement process. The sheets are reviewed at the next session.

The third major goal of stress management, making choices about coping strategies, is intensively discussed in Session 6. Participants first learn to classify their coping responses as either problem focused or emotion focused. They are encouraged to discuss examples of situations in which they commonly use these strategies. Participants then learn that both categories of coping strategies include productive (and usually direct) or nonproductive (and usually indirect) methods. They then discuss recent stressful situations in which they have used these methods. During the subsequent week, participants monitor any stressful situations that occur, their automatic thoughts and rational thought replacements (if applicable), and the coping strategies they used to deal with the stressor. Each strategy is categorized as problem focused or emotion focused and productive or nonproductive. Participants also learn that just as coping responses can be categorized, so can different aspects of stressful situations. Using the coping theory developed by Folkman and Lazarus (1980) and more recently adapted to psychosocial interventions by Folkman et al. (1991), we ask participants to identify the controllable and uncontrollable aspects of stressful situations and then match problem-focused productive strategies with controllable aspects of stressors and emotion-focused productive strategies with uncontrollable aspects. Participants are then given examples of several breast cancer–related stressors. They are asked to complete an exercise wherein they identify the controllable and uncontrollable aspects of the stressor, list possible productive problem-focused and emotion-focused coping responses, and finally match the most appropriate coping response with the stressor aspect being identified. During the subsequent week, participants monitor stressful events in their lives and complete a similar analysis on self-monitoring sheets that they bring back to the next group meeting.

The final goal of stress management, better use of resources to help deal with stressors, is accomplished in three sessions. We have reasoned that because interpersonal conflict can be a key obstacle to accessing coping resources, teaching group members interpersonal conflict resolution skills might be particularly effective in enhancing their ability to use such resources. During Session 7, participants are encouraged to discuss the meaning of social support in their lives. They discuss their most valuable social relationships, the people who have been the most supportive in their lives, and the ways in which they provide support to others. They learn that social support can exist in many forms, ranging from informational support (e.g., getting advice) to emotional support (e.g., love and nurturance). Next, participants are allowed to discuss their own obstacles to obtaining and maintaining a support network and the ways in which breast cancer has played a role in this process. Finally, they apply CBSM techniques learned during the B-SMART program to address their social support obstacles. This portion of the program, which was discussed previously, involves challenging cognitive appraisals involved in withdrawal and isolation, modifying coping strategies for accessing social support, and reevaluating the situation after making coping changes.

In Session 8, participants get intensive training in anger management. They complete exercises designed to increase their awareness of the unique ways in which they experience and express angry feelings and the role anger plays in their lives. Next, participants identify personal anger triggers and some of the physical consequences of their anger. Two common anger pathways are highlighted in this session—explosive anger and stuffing anger. During the explosive anger discussion, participants learn to identify and slow down the automatic thoughts that precede angry outbursts, label the corresponding cognitive distortions (e.g., black-and-white thinking), and challenge and replace the distortions as necessary with more rational thoughts (i.e., appraisals). A similar discussion addresses stuffing anger. Participants complete several exercises designed to demonstrate examples of each type of anger pathway. During the subsequent week, they are asked to monitor anger-inducing situations, including their physical responses to the situations, accompanying self-talk (appraisals), and possible alternative responses. These observations are recorded on sheets provided in the *Participant's Workbook*.

During the next session (Session 9), participants learn to communicate assertively. Group leaders begin this session by introducing participants to four communication styles—aggressive, passive, passive–aggressive, and assertive—and highlight the advantages and disadvantages of each. The members then learn ways assertiveness decreases stress and the reason it is the most efficient means of communicating. During in-session role-playing, participants learn to identify each type of communication style in scenarios that are listed in their *Participant's Workbook*. After they have sharpened their skills in detecting each of the different communication styles, participants discuss some of their personal barriers to behaving assertively (e.g., fear of rejection, a mistaken sense of responsibility and their own rights) and how they can overcome these barriers. Participants then complete exercises on ways to send assertive messages. During the subsequent week, they are asked to monitor the occurrence of stressful situations and their accompanying automatic thoughts and emotions, as well as the style of communication that they used with the people involved in the situations. Finally, members are asked to think of an alternative communication style that they could have used. Participants use the monitoring sheets in their *Participant's Workbook* to assess any interpersonal stressors that occur during the week; they present the sheets to their group leaders at the final session.

At this point, participants are also encouraged to integrate the techniques they learned in the anger management and assertiveness training sessions to increase their efficiency at enhancing their social network. The B-SMART program is a progressive and structured program that introduces the simple concepts and exercises underlying the use of relaxation-based and stress management techniques. The relaxation-based techniques progress from simpler muscle relaxation exercises to more complex blends of guided imagery with deep breathing, autogenics, and meditation. The stress management techniques progress from simpler awareness-aising exercises to more complex cognitive–behavioral techniques such as cognitive restructuring, coping skills training, anger management, and assertiveness skills. The program progresses not only from simple to more complex strategies but also (in accordance with our stress management theory) from more cognitive activities (e.g., making appraisals), to behavioral activities (e.g., coping), to interpersonal activities (expressing anger, communicating assertively, using social support).

MAINTENANCE SESSIONS

To maintain intervention gains, facilitators of the program may chose to use a regular follow-up protocol. After the program ends, B-SMART participants may be scheduled for monthly maintenance sessions so that they can (a) receive feedback and reinforcement for treatment gains and adherence, (b) turn in their completed weekly self-monitoring cards and records of cognitive responses to stressors, and (c) receive a 1-month supply of blank cards and thought-monitoring sheets. During the maintenance sessions, participants are encouraged to discuss successful and unsuccessful experiences using the CBSM techniques and discuss obstacles to fitting the relaxation exercises into their daily routines. Based on previous relapse prevention interventions with others (Roffman, Beadnell, & Gordon, 1991), we have incorporated some of the following components in these maintenance sessions: (a) identification of high-risk factors (e.g., emotional factors) for reverting to use of extreme stress responses, (b) identification of environmental cues for relapse (e.g., people, places, certain times of day), (c) identification of positive expectations for substance use, (d) instruction on cognitive strategies (e.g., self-talk) and behavioral strategies (e.g., self-monitoring), and (e) encouragement for

CBSM strategies that seem to be the most effective. These strategies have been derived from studies of adherence to various behavioral interventions (Brownell, Marlatt, Lichenstein, & Wilson, 1986; Dishman & Ickes, 1981; Marlatt & George, 1989).

We have used monthly maintenance sessions after the completion of our 10-week program and found that participants were eager to attend such meetings. At these sessions, they are encouraged to do the following:

- Describe the recent stressors they have experienced and the degree to which they have been able to use CBSM strategies to handle them
- Describe alternative coping strategies they have developed and factors that seem to facilitate or obstruct their ability to cope successfully with stressors
- Monitor their perceived stress levels and relaxation practice frequency on a weekly basis and record this information on monitoring cards or sheets that are turned in at each maintenance session

At the end of the 6-month maintenance period, group facilitators can give group members the opportunity to continue meeting on a monthly basis and allow one of the group leaders to conduct these groups (which are structured as open groups). This procedure has been used in studies of psychosocial interventions for patients with cancer and those with other types of medical problems (Fawzy, Kemeny, et al., 1990). We also refer participants to local support organizations that have ongoing groups for women with breast cancer. Initial results from these maintenance sessions indicate that the participants are using their newly learned cognitive restructuring techniques, assertiveness skills, and relaxation exercises; are improving their personal relationships and experiencing less perceived stress; and are enjoying the opportunity to talk with others about their frustrations and progress in using these strategies.

Intervention and Training Materials

THERAPIST'S MANUAL

As indicated in the outline for each weekly session, each session is organized into relaxation and imagery material and stress management material. The relaxation and imagery material includes a brief description of the rationale for each specific relaxation technique (e.g., seven-muscle-group PMR) or imagery-related technique (e.g., autogenics with guided

Materials for Implementing Intervention Sessions

We have developed several types of material for conducting the B-SMART program, and they are included in the *Therapist's Manual* and the *Participant's Workbook*. Briefly, the *Therapist's Manual* contains information necessary to introduce group leaders from a wide variety of backgrounds and training experiences to the use of CBSM techniques with patients with breast cancer. The manual is divided into 10 modules that coincide with the 10 weekly sessions of the B-SMART program. Each module contains an outline of the supplies needed for the session and a summary of the techniques and exercises being introduced. The outline of techniques and exercises is subdivided into those concerning relaxation and imagery and those concerning stress management activities. However, the most important sections of the manual are those containing the didactic material.

imagery). The descriptions are followed by a detailed description of the steps involved in preparing participants for the relaxation induction and the script for the specific technique. The manual also provides discussion questions for participants to answer after they have completed the exercise. Like the relaxation material, the stress management material includes a description of the rationale for using the specific stress management techniques, such as cognitive restructuring, coping skills, assertive communication, and anger management. The material also describes ways to help group members handle minor daily stressors and more serious and chronic stressors emanating from breast cancer. The manual includes several illustrations designed to facilitate the presentation of the material; they can be used in handouts or overhead transparencies. In any given session, the description of the rationale for a stress management technique is either accompanied or followed by an in-session written or role-play exercise designed to raise participants' awareness of some aspect of stress responses and their sequelae that are particularly relevant to the stress management technique being introduced that week.

PARTICIPANT'S WORKBOOK

The *Participant's Workbook* is designed to provide group members with an overview of the B-SMART program, detailed summaries of the rationale for and content of each of the 10 stress management sessions, and several exercises that can be used between the weekly group meetings. The overview of the program orients participants to our general expectations about their involvement in the stress management process, emphasizes the importance of practicing out-of-session activities, and reviews some of the basic rules of the group sessions (e.g., confidentiality). Similar to the *Therapist's Manual*, the *Participant's Workbook* is divided into 10 modules that coincide with the 10 weekly sessions of the B-SMART program. In fact, the workbook has been designed to correspond with the manual; group leaders are instructed to incorporate actual workbook sections into certain activities conducted in the group sessions. All participants should bring their workbooks to every session.

The *Participant's Workbook* contains extensive information about the stress management techniques learned at the group meetings. Beginning in Module 1, the workbook provides activities designed to raise participants' awareness of subtle stress-processing steps (e.g., asking participants to list their personal physical and emotional symptoms of stress), and the activities are used to catalyze group discussions. In subsequent sessions, the workbook provides at least one activity per session that is designed to increase participants' awareness of different subtle psychological phenomena such as stress responses, automatic thoughts, and cognitive distortions; emotion-focused vs. problem-focused coping strategies; anger expression patterns and underlying cognitive processes; assertive behaviors and their interpersonal consequences; and the positive and negative elements of their social networks . All of these activities are facilitated by group leaders in the weekly sessions through written exercises and behavioral role-playing.

In addition to these in-session activities, each workbook session contains a take-home activity designed to help individuals practice applying their newly learned CBSM techniques to stressors and events that occur in their everyday lives. In the initial stages of the program, these activities involve asking participants to record the thoughts, feelings, and physical sensations associated with stressful events. This process helps increase their awareness of their characteristic responses. As members proceed through the program, these take-home activities increase in complexity and involve recording (a) cognitive distortions and the rational thoughts used to replace them, (b) maladaptive coping strategies and alternative strategies used to replace them, (c) inappropriate anger responses and alternative, more balanced responses used to replace them, and (d) passive, indirect communication and more assertive communication used to replace it. Each of these activities is completed on a Stress Monitoring Sheet at the end of each workbook session. Participants complete these activities during the week and discuss them at the beginning of the stress management portion of each weekly meeting.

In each workbook module, participants are provided with a synopsis of the relaxation and guided imagery technique learned that week. Although participants learn the actual relaxation and imagery techniques in the group sessions, the workbook modules include a summary of the steps used to implement the technique. In addition, the workbook contains a self-monitoring form that participants use to monitor the frequency of their relaxation exercise practice sessions. This form can be reproduced as a full-size form or as a wallet-size card that can be given to participants in packets of seven at each weekly meeting. The forms are turned in each week. Group leaders can use the information to praise group members for regular practice or to identify individuals who may need extra help organizing their schedules for their relaxation practice. The *Therapist's Manual* and the *Participant's Workbook* are the backbone of the B-SMART program and should be used together in the program's implementation.

TRAINING GROUP LEADERS

During the developmental and field trial stages of the B-SMART program, we used advanced clinical health psychology graduate students, postdoctoral fellows, and licensed clinical psychologists to conduct the group sessions. Although the program has never been tested with other health care professionals (e.g., nurses, licensed clinical social workers), the *Therapist's Manual* has been designed to be an appropriate guide for any professional with prior group therapy and mental health training experience. In some cases, non–mental health care professionals who have had extensive experience in conducting focused patient support groups may also be able to implement the program with relative ease. We recommend that all prospective group leaders complete a training sequence, guided by the manual and conducted for a 10-week period, before implementing the program. The training can be enhanced with intensive in-class training in PMR, guided imagery, deep breathing, autogenics, meditation, cognitive restructuring, coping skills, anger management, and assertiveness. Some group leaders may want to enhance these basic readings by exploring more specialized research on topics such as counseling issues in patients with cancer, psychosocial and sociocultural factors associated with medical diseases and treatments, relaxation-based techniques, cognitive therapy, anger management, assertion training, and group therapy process issues (e.g., Beck & Emery, 1979; Bernstein & Borkovec, 1973; Greer et al., 1992; Hersen et al., 1973; Spira, 1997; Yalom & Greaves, 1977). One major component that needs to be incorporated into training is addressing the group leaders' own fears about and vulnerabilities related to cancer. This issue is most effectively handled during the supervisory process. (The process is discussed using case examples in chapter 4.)

In our studies of the B-SMART program conducted to date, all sessions were audiotaped or videotaped (with participants' informed consent), and the tapes were reviewed by two licensed mental health professionals on a weekly basis. This protocol was necessary for us to standardize the research environment while evaluating the program. The use of the B-SMART program in clinical settings would be monitored by different methods. For instance, clinicians supervising subordinates who are leading the B-SMART groups or are consulting with other allied health professionals (e.g., nurses, social case workers) who are conducting the sessions should meet with the group leaders on a weekly basis to review each session's events. Adherence to the weekly sessions (as outlined in the treatment manual) can be monitored through these weekly face-to-face supervision meetings. Clinicians who use the program may have other specific ways to ensure the fidelity of the intervention. It is important to stress that although several of the CBSM techniques constituting the program may be used by patients to build their interpersonal skills, they are all designed to be taught and reviewed in a group format under the guidance of trained group leaders. Therefore, the program is far more than a collection of self-help techniques.

Implementing the B-SMART Program | 4

Tailoring the B-SMART Program

The B-SMART program was developed for women with breast cancer in various stages of disease and treatment, ranging from the initial diagnosis stage to the adjuvant therapy stage to the postadjuvant therapy period. Women with metastatic breast cancer may benefit more from the emotional support offered by this program than from the actual CBSM techniques that they learn. The program can be tailored to women with metastatic breast cancer by increasing the focus on social ties and group sharing and decreasing the focus on all of the specific stress reduction techniques. To date, we have very little information about the effectiveness of this program for men and women dealing with other cancers because most of the initial studies were focused on women with breast cancer. We are currently examining the effectiveness of programs like B-SMART for women at risk for cervical cancer, men with early-stage prostate cancer, and men and women with chronic medical conditions such as HIV infection and AIDS, chronic fatigue syndrome, and cardiovascular disease. These studies will address some of the unanswered questions concerning the generalizability of the program. A current major project

---

This chapter was written in collaboration with Roselyn G. Smith. At the time of this writing, Roselyn G. Smith was a doctoral student in the Department of Psychology. Her research was conducted primarily with breast cancer patients, and she was co-therapist for several B-SMART groups during her tenure.

involves translating these programs into Spanish so that they can be useful for the growing population of monolingual, Spanish-speaking people living in the major metropolitan regions of the United States.

General Challenges to Using the Program

Like creators of any intervention based on a manual, we have no way to anticipate or account for the range of individual responses to diagnosis and treatment for breast cancer that group members will have, nor can we fully anticipate the multiple group dynamics that will be involved. We have three goals in this chapter. First, we describe some of the more common issues and dynamics in various groups that we have observed while using the B-SMART intervention. Second, we present commentaries from B-SMART participants at various stages of the intervention, focusing on their thoughts about the impact of the intervention as the 10-week program concluded and at 3-, 6-, or 12-month follow-ups. In addition, the chapter discusses some common issues encountered by group leaders, such as countertransference issues and feelings that can result from working with patients with breast cancer. Specific case examples are used. Names and other potentially identifying characteristics have been altered for confidentiality.

In most groups, the first two sessions successfully accomplished the first goal of the intervention: raising participants' awareness of stress in their lives. The intervention is designed to progress from a state of increased stress awareness toward understanding, identification, and replacement of the cognitive components that unnecessarily contribute to stress responses. The stress awareness step is critical and should be carefully monitored. If group members are not warned that they may actually feel more stressed as a result of their newfound awareness, they may become even more distressed, thinking that they have actually increased their stress level rather than their stress awareness level. The group leaders should prepare group members for this phenomenon with a statement such as the following:

> Occasionally when people become involved with a group like this, they actually feel more stressed out in the beginning. We want you to be aware that part of the work we are doing here is designed to raise your awareness of your own stress levels by drawing your attention to your physical manifestations of stress and your subjective emotional experiences. You shouldn't be surprised if as you become more aware of how stress is functioning in your life, you feel a little more stressed at first.

During the first few weeks, group members tend to compare their treatments, which can increase their stress as well. They often become focused on chemotherapy regimens, comparing surgical procedures, and discussing other differences in treatment decisions. Group members may begin to question their treatment choices. The solution is to be aware of and address this group dynamic. Listen very carefully for any mention of treatment issues, and then emphasize that every person's experience with breast cancer is unique. Explain that cancer is really a composite of physiological events, so the relative individuality of the disease drives the treatment recommendations made by medical professionals.

Group leaders can mitigate second-guessing about medical decisions by telling group members who are uncomfortable with their treatment regimens to speak with their doctors or get second and third opinions from qualified professionals. Techniques for discussing these types of issues with medical professionals are not specifically addressed until the ninth session, which involves assertiveness training. The point of addressing treatment comparisons early in the program is to prevent the development of additional stress. If treatment comparisons do begin, they can be used as examples of cognitive distortions when the concept is discussed in Session 3. For example, during Session 3, the group leader can recall previous discussions about treatments:

> Remember when you were discussing the differences in your treatments? Some of you may have had thoughts such as, "My doctor is giving me a type of chemotherapy that no one else in the group is getting. Maybe this means my cancer is worse than theirs." Which types of cognitive distortions were involved in this thought pattern?

The answer would include catastrophic thinking and perhaps "should" statements, and the snowball effect.

Dealing With Resistance

At least one participant per group questions or denies the personal relevance of certain parts of the intervention. This type of resistance typically arises in response to one of four issues: (a) the necessity of structured relaxation practice, (b) recognition of personal cognitive distortions, (c) acceptance of the concept that anger is adaptive in certain situations (because many participants want to deny the existence and use of anger), and (d) discomfort with communicating assertively. Knowing that resistance is likely to be encountered in one or more of these four areas

Members Who Blame Themselves

One stress-increasing thought we have seen develop within and across groups is the idea that group members have caused their cancer. Members may make statements such as, "My life has been so stressful for the last few years. Somewhere deep down inside, I knew something like his would happen. If only I had changed my life earlier." We intervene at the first sign of these attributions with a heavy dose of psychoeducation. We clarify that although everyone intuitively knows that stress is unhealthy, even scientists and medical doctors do not know exactly how it affects the progression of diseases such as cancer. We continue by explaining to group members that blaming themselves for their breast cancer can induce more stress and that they should be applauded for deciding to learn some new ways to handle stress.

may help the group leaders develop strategies in advance to effectively address these issues when they arise.

RESISTANCE TO RELAXATION

Resistance to structured relaxation has manifested in numerous ways during the years. Statements ranging from, "I can't breathe deeply because I gag when I try," to "Relaxation doesn't work for me," to "I can't relax at home because I fall asleep," are common. Responses to these statements should focus on helping members incorporate the relaxation techniques in any way possible. In other words, if a participant gags when she takes deep breaths or focuses on her breathing, give her permission to modify the deep breathing until it is comfortable for her. Some women are not comfortable stretching out on mats or futons on the floor. Let them sit in their chairs, prop their feet up, or sit with their feet comfortably stretched out in front of them. The point is that group members who are uncomfortable with what they are being asked to do are likely to focus on those feelings and derive no benefit from the relaxation exercise. In addition, reinforce all attempts to relax, even if they include approaches not mentioned in our manual. For example, if someone is not using the relaxation exercises but is taking yoga classes, acknowledge the effort and suggest that the participant use one of the relaxation techniques we offer (e.g. guided imagery) at the end of their yoga practice during the meditation. One woman initially reported that although she had not been practicing the relaxation exercise at home, she was able to use progressive muscle relaxation (PMR) to relax her shoulders at work after a particularly stressful interaction with her boss.

Eventually, we tie in the aspects of given techniques participants like to one or more of the exercises we offer and emphasize the similarities. When a participant continues to resist—does not practice during the week or makes statements about not feeling relaxed during an in-session exercise—we take a more direct approach. We revisit the rationale behind relaxation and explore possible deterrents (and their solutions) to home relaxation practice. We also give feedback about how the person looked and behaved during the in-session relaxation exercise. For example, statements such as, "I noticed that 10 minutes into the relaxation exercise, you actually were taking very deep breaths," have helped to dispel qualms about gagging or choking when focusing on breathing. The statement, "You say the relaxation didn't work for you this time, but at one point I noticed how relaxed your arms and legs were and how peaceful you looked," is another way to gently challenge the "I can't relax" statement.

Some participants who have experienced previous trauma or who have repressed the intensity of anxiety they are feeling in response to their diagnosis and treatment experience substantial feelings of resistance or even an abreaction during relaxation exercises. If this occurs, the group leader who is monitoring the relaxation session (not the one leading the relaxation session) goes to the individuals and speaks to them gently, possibly touching their shoulder. It is critical to process what happened after the relaxation exercise ends. Normalizing the response with a statement such as, "Sometimes this kind of reaction just happens," may significantly mitigate additional distress that could develop when these members try to relax outside of the session.

Although in this CBSM group setting we do not recommend completely addressing the ramifications of previous traumatic experiences, it is imperative to understand that some individuals have used coping strategies that have forced them to remain alert and vigilant and to repress distressing thoughts or feelings. For example, if someone is deeply traumatized by the loss of one or both breasts and is not ready to acknowledge the impact of the experience, remaining in a heightened state of arousal may keep the intensity of the experience at bay until she is ready to process it. Ultimately, we want to address the cognitions and resulting emotions surrounding the experience to minimize its power to induce distress. Relaxation helps facilitate this process. One option is to directly acknowledge that some people use this type of coping to handle overwhelming emotions. In other words, addressing the coping style being used rather than the emotion the coping is ameliorating may be safer than plowing ahead with a discussion of the fears and loss associated with double mastectomy or a previous trauma.

COGNITIVE DISTORTIONS? NOT ME!

Participants may also resist when the concept of cognitive distortions is introduced. Some people so strongly feel the need to be right that even considering the possibility their thoughts could be inaccurate is threatening. We have addressed this common response in numerous ways, and many of the methods are included as exercises in the manual. The important point to remember, regardless of the exercise chosen (e.g., "Imagine a Person You Are Having Trouble With. Now Imagine Someone You Love," "Lemon Imagery"), is that the group members' thoughts about an undesirable person lead to their anger, frustration, dislike, or disgust. Similarly, it is their thoughts about people they love that lead to feelings of warmth or a smile. In the Lemon Imagery exercise, we make the point that thoughts are even powerful enough to make people salivate when they are imaging a lemon! This point cannot be made too strongly or reinforced too frequently. During one B-SMART program, a group leader reminded a participant who became angry when thinking of a friend, "We didn't bring him into the room and let him make you feel that way. Your thoughts about him created the feelings."

It is usually necessary to reemphasize the link between certain types of distortions and the specific feelings they stimulate. However, it is very powerful to listen to a participant's comments, ask the person permission to repeat something said, and then ask other members of the group, "Which categories of distortions might be involved in what she just said?" Sometimes the other group members will leap to the defense of the group member whose thoughts are being examined. Regardless, the group leaders should not be swayed and should still firmly and gently identify and explain the potential distortion. We do not argue with the group members—rather, we state that a given statement sounds like it could be a distortion but do not insist that everyone has to agree with the assessment.

ANGER IS BAD

Discomfort with and denial of anger may be evident in statements such as, "Since I've been diagnosed with breast cancer, I don't feel angry any more." Resistance may manifest as direct opposition to the assertion that anger can be an adaptive and useful emotion. Distinguishing (repeatedly if necessary) between the emotion of anger and how it often manifests behaviorally is a key step. When the "I'm no longer angry" issue surfaces early in the intervention, we assure participants that we will address anger more fully in the later anger management session (Session 8). An integral exercise in the anger management session—an exercise that is usually a very powerful tool—asks participants to consider how each of their parents or other significant childhood figures dealt with anger. Once the exercise is completed, individuals who are reluctant to acknowledge the adaptability of anger may spontaneously realize that they learned to fear anger because of the behaviors they associate with it. Others may need direct intervention in the form of empathic statements such as, "It is easy to understand why you feel that anger serves no good purpose when you saw it expressed in such painful and confusing ways." It is helpful to explain that anger is often terribly uncomfortable because most people are never given the tools to use it effectively.

RESISTANCE TO ASSERTIVENESS

Assertiveness is "the tool" most of people were not given when they were learning how to communicate their needs, anger, and other emotions. Interestingly, the concept of assertiveness may be met with resistance by members who freely but aggressively express their anger, those who are passive–aggressive in their expression of anger, and those who are more passive (i.e., who "stuff") their anger. In addition, assertiveness and aggressiveness are often confused. By this point in the B-SMART program (Session 9), most group members know that their group leaders will deal quite directly with them when necessary. We try to identify members' typical communication styles while keeping in mind the nature of our rapport with them and their ability to handle direct comments. The case study example of Francesca and Louise, described later in this chapter, demonstrates how this can be accomplished.

Finally, on an anecdotal basis, a consensus seems to exist among breast cancer patients that since their diagnosis, they no longer feel angry about things that used to upset them. For some patients, the need to cope with the disease probably directs emotional resources away from everyday annoyances so that they can focus on treatment decisions and existential concerns. We caution women in our groups that they should not assume that these new priorities (e.g., changes in what constitutes something worthy of anger) will last. We tell them that previous annoyances are likely to resurface and that we address anger in the intervention because it is a normal and adaptive response to some stimuli. We also let them know that we are explaining this so that they do not become disappointed when they find themselves feeling angry again. We do not want them to think that feelings of anger or annoyance constitute some kind of spiritual or moral decline from a previously enlightened position. Instead, we ask them to acknowledge their anger—past and present—and give them tools for working with it. These and other issues are clarified in the following case study examples.

Case Studies

SHIRLEY: SHAPING A MEMBER'S BEHAVIOR TO FACILITATE THE GROUP PROCESS

Communication styles of individual group members may have to be addressed during intervention to help make the group intervention successful. Otherwise, the behavior of a group member who is lacking in social skills or is insensitive to others may impede the group process. One of our former participants, Shirley, comes to mind. Shirley was a divorced woman in her early 40s who worked as a manager in a library at a local university. She reported having few friends her own age and relied primarily on her older mother and father and their friends for social support.

Shirley primarily disclosed work-related information and did so somewhat pedantically, focusing on the minutiae of her somewhat tedious routine. When other group members disclosed more personal information, Shirley would respond in one of two ways. Initially, she tried to analyze their comments and feelings in ways that were occasionally accurate but were insensitive and seemed to be projections of her own thoughts and feelings. On other occasions, Shirley would direct discussions away from emotionally laden topics by launching into an account of a somewhat tangential topic or making comparisons to her own experiences in ways that ended the conversation. For example, when one group member was grappling with her breast cancer diagnosis and the resulting complex and difficult feelings about her young children, Shirley stated, "Well, it seems to me that your husband isn't helping you enough. That happened to me with my ex-husband. He was only concerned about himself, and I am glad he isn't here while I am dealing with breast cancer." Not only was her assessment of the prevailing issue completely off track, it directed the discussion away from a very important disclosure by another group member.

Eventually, group members displayed signs of annoyance with Shirley any time she began to speak, even when her comments were salient. The group leaders decided that direct intervention was needed to help Shirley develop appropriate social skills, prevent the group from ostracizing her, and keep the group climate conducive to an open exchange of ideas. While continuing to introduce and work with the cognitive–behavioral–based intervention, the group leaders mentioned Shirley's apparent discomfort with emotionally laden topics. In addition, when Shirley would make a statement implying the superiority of her approach to treatment or other decisions, one of the group leaders would reply, "So, that is the decision you made for yourself based on your set of circumstances. Can you see how someone else might make a different decision?" The group members then started gently confronting Shirley and identifying differences between their situations and hers. The group leaders also began making very direct comments to Shirley when she attempted to truncate another group member's disclosure. One would hold a hand up in her direction and say, "Excuse me, Shirley. I am interested in what you have to say, but right now I would like to hear this group member finish her thoughts." Within two sessions of using this very intentional approach, Shirley began monitoring her own interactions, listening to other group members, minimizing interpretations and comparisons, and disclosing more personal issues. She eventually began talking about the intervention goals and trying to understand how she was contributing to stress in her life.

At the end of the 10 weeks, Shirley thanked the group leaders for including her in the group, stating, "I always thought I dealt with things in a competent, professional manner and that this approach could be used to cope with my breast cancer. What I was missing was a way to be comfortable with feelings, especially scary ones. I know I still need to work on it, but now I understand that emotion-focused coping is just as important as problem-focused coping, especially if some aspects of a stressor are uncontrollable."

CARMEN: CONFRONTING EXISTENTIAL ISSUES

Our own research on the prevailing concerns of patients with breast cancer has revealed that existential concerns contribute heavily to the distress associated with the disease (Spencer et al., 1999). The emotional experience associated with a life-threatening disease may indeed involve cognitive distortions, but the experience is based in reality. Our team has grappled with how best to address patients' existential issues, which usually manifest as concerns about not being able to live out their life with their partner or not being able to live to see their small children grow into adulthood. After hours of evaluation and deliberation, we determined that given the stated and implied goals of the intervention (i.e., not only to provide techniques for managing stress but also to also promote positive growth from the breast cancer experience), we would be remiss in trying to cognitively challenge perceived existential threats. Indeed, it is our belief that the existential aspects of dealing with the disease provide the motivation to pursue life changes and seek out the positive as patients progress through their treatment and into the post-treatment period. Group leaders have many opportunities to educate participants about the identification and replacement of cognitive distortions. Rather than using substantial existential concerns to build these skills, we recommend using less poignant situations to introduce and solidify the cognitive approach.

Carmen joined the B-SMART clinical outcome trials shortly after surgery. She was 35 years old and had a ready smile and quick wit—she quickly became the darling of the group. She was the mother of a 5-year-old boy and a 2-year-old girl. She and her husband were both professionals, and she reported that their relationship was strong and supportive. Carmen often entertained the group with humorous accounts of her life, after which tears would occasionally well up in her eyes. The group leaders noticed that the tears always followed stories of her children. A group leader asked, "What are your tears trying to say?" Carmen responded that she felt awful her children had to see her so sick and going bald from the chemotherapy.

During the anger management session (Session 8), Carmen reported that she had been very angry with her husband during the previous week. He had not seemed concerned enough about an accident involving their son. The accident involved a family pet, which the husband allowed to live in the house. Carmen was furious that the husband "chose the pet over the child." She used this situation to try to identify possible cognitive distortions associated with her anger. She discovered the she was confused by the intensity of her reaction because the situation—in her opinion—was really not that serious. The group members rallied around her, supporting her angry feelings toward her husband. She responded by stating her husband was really a great guy and that she did not understand why the event had made her so angry. One of the group leaders used this opportunity to tell Carmen that every time she had become upset in a group session, her children were being discussed. Carmen acknowledged that the group leader was right. She revealed that what she was really concerned about was whether her husband would be able to care for the children by himself if she died.

The incident with the pet allowed her to acknowledge her fear of dying from breast cancer and her subsequent feelings of profound loss involving the children. She also said that having breast cancer felt like a loss of innocence as far as her health was concerned. The group leaders did not challenge her when she said she might die, challenge her concerns about her children, or challenge her difficult feelings about no longer being immune to disease. Rather, they used "softening" (a coping technique presented in Session 5) to process her painful emotions and empathized with how difficult it must be to be a mother of young children and have the disease. In the B-SMART model, coping is developed on the premise that some aspects of stressors are controllable, and some are uncontrollable. People often have the most success coping with controllable aspects by using problem-focused strategies, whereas emotion-focused strategies are often best for uncontrollable aspects (see specific sessions for descriptions). After an accurate assessment of cognitive distortions and problem-focused and emotion-focused strategy development, group members will still have difficult feelings remaining, such as those involving their mortality. At this point, softening, accepting, or "sitting with" their feelings is encouraged. Our hope is that by allowing the feelings to exist, group members can learn to tolerate the existence of the feelings.

In subsequent sessions, the group leaders challenged Carmen's approaches to asserting herself with family members. She responded splendidly and used some new approaches with the "most difficult" member of her family. During one session, Carmen discussed a recent interaction with this difficult family member: "She was really nice to me when I explained that sometimes I just don't want to talk about the cancer. She told me that she just wanted to be there for me and didn't know how— so I told her how she could best help me, and she was really happy. I had built up fears about offending her and therefore the rest of the family, and my fears didn't come true. It makes me wonder if I am using that kind of distorted thinking in other areas of my life."

Carmen's case study provides an excellent opportunity to examine the fine line that exists between cognitive distortions and poignant existential issues. In Carmen's case, it would have been fairly easy (and perhaps more comfortable for the group leaders) to point out the obvious distortions in her thoughts. She was "catastrophizing," "minimizing the positive," and even "mind reading" in her interaction with her husband. The group leaders made the decision to support her as she confronted her own mortality. Their decision was perhaps based equally on knowledge of research on existential phenomena in people with cancer, keen observations of Carmen's disclosure patterns in the previous weeks, and sound clinical judgment. Group members looked to Carmen for ready smiles and reassurance. She was a confident woman who felt compelled to hide her fears from her family and friends. Perhaps that was her greatest distortion of all—thinking she could not express her fears about death to those closest to her. In essence, she was afraid to use her social support network. The group allowed her fears to surface, be acknowledged, and be contained. When the program is over, it becomes a model for using social support.

It is our contention that being afraid of dying from cancer is not a distorted thought. It is an understandable response to a life-threatening disease about which far too little is known. Our premise, which is based on research that preceded the development of B-SMART and anecdotal information garnered during years of working with B-SMART groups, is that people with cancer must acknowledge and work through the associated existential issues even as they are trying to effectively manage stress. Although no specific session is dedicated to addressing existential issues, from the very first session, group leaders need to be attuned to the existential overtones and ready to address issues of mortality.

Each group usually has at least one person who is comfortable disclosing personal information and is open and willing to receive the didactic information and incorporate it into her disclosures. Carmen was this person in her group. These participants are relatively easy to work with and a boon to the group and group leaders. It can become tempting to rely on those group members to openly embrace the material, generate discussions, and prevent awkward silences or even challenges to the material and group leaders. Conversely, participants who remain quiet, have an "I'm handling this just fine, thank you" attitude, or question the program material are challenging for group leaders. If these situations are not resolved, countertransference issues may emerge. In group leaders' desire to have enough time to check in with the group, discuss the weekly topic, check homework, and introduce a new relaxation technique, it is understandable that they may be drawn toward group members who make the job a little easier. Conversely, more difficult group members can create resistances or "pull for" rejection, so it takes a bit more effort from the group leaders to connect with them. In the following three case studies, the participation of the each of the group members—Estelle, Roxanne, and Allison—may have been improved if the group leaders had spent a little more time working with them in the group sessions or had approached them differently.

ESTELLE: THE RESERVED GROUP MEMBER

Estelle was a 38-year-old woman who was married to a firefighter and worked as a secretary in the fire department. She had a high school education and some formal secretarial and computer training. She was less educated and in a less prestigious job than the other members in her group. Estelle was very quiet and disclosed very little in the first five or six sessions. When she started to disclose information in later sessions, she would couch her stories in such as way that implied she had no stress in her life at all. The group leaders felt uncomfortable pressuring Estelle to speak, openly discussing her discomfort when speaking within the group, and pushing her to admit that she had stressors. They were worried that by making her speak they would destroy her self-esteem and force her to reveal socioeconomic and educational information that she would have considered embarrassing.

Approximately halfway through the 10-week intervention, the group leaders decided to start calling on Estelle to share her homework. This seemed to be a safe and relatively unobtrusive way to help her begin sharing. She could maintain as much control as she needed but be more involved in the group discussions. Estelle seemed very uncomfortable at first but was able to accurately apply the material to some situations in her life. Group leaders and group members reinforced her for sharing, and she began to establish a friendship with another member. During Session 7 (the social support session), Estelle was ready to share. She recounted a very difficult interaction with her daughter, who was in her early 20s. She asked her daughter for help but instead of helping, the daughter created a situation that led to more work for Estelle, who was experiencing some extremely uncomfortable reactions to her chemotherapy. In Sessions 8 and 9, Estelle was ill with opportunistic respiratory infections, and it was clear that it required much effort just to attend the group meetings. Estelle let the group leaders know that she could not go any further in her disclosure by ceasing to do her homework or at least telling the group leaders this was the case.

Perhaps the group leaders could have thought of ways for Estelle to share earlier in the intervention. In addition, they made assumptions about why she was not speaking. Although Estelle's behavior appeared to be that of someone who was anxious in a group setting, the group leaders did not actually know the origin of that discomfort. They will never know what would have happened if they had simply asked her to share her homework examples earlier in the program.

ROXANNE: THE SUPERCOPER

Some group members think that the experience of breast cancer and treatment should not disrupt their lives on any level. They think they must continue to be supermoms, superemployees, superhostesses, and superpartners. In the extreme, these "supercopers" are the ones who are at risk for dropping out after the first or second session. They begin to become aware that they are incredibly stressed because they are unable to tolerate imperfection in any aspect of their lives. Supercopers who remain in the program often emphasize that they are just fine, are keeping up with all of the demands of their busy lives, and know the "right" way to cope—which is to stay busy and ignore the effects of having breast cancer and undergoing treatment.

Various group members defend this position with different levels of intensity. One former group member, Roxanne, is a wonderful example of a supercoper who was able to gain a new perspective and process some of her distress.

Roxanne was in her mid 50s and managed her husband's law office. She was always well dressed, was very polite, and engaged in the group discussions and process in a supportive but guarded manner. Early in the program, she reported that she had incorporated the relaxation tapes into her daily routine and was trying different ones. Around Session 4 or 5, Roxanne listened to the relaxation exercise that was to be presented in Session 10—the last of the B-SMART program. The exercise invites group members to "leave something behind" in a crystal box on a deserted beach. The exercise is intended to help group members have closure as the group ends and to make choices about what thoughts and behaviors they would like to permanently leave behind.

Roxanne reported that as she was invited to leave something in the box, she started to cry. She experienced intense feelings of loss. She remained relaxed as she questioned herself about what she had lost, and the answer came to her—she had lost her breasts. She thought she had accepted the loss of her breasts after her double mastectomy, but she discovered that powerful feelings remained. In her mind, she placed the breasts into the crystal box, mourned, and told them good-bye. When she talked about this experience in the session, she did so with little emotion and maintained a composed, professional manner. The other group members remained silent. The group leaders felt somewhat taken aback at this "supercoper's" disclosure of such a profound and vulnerable experience. They too had become accustomed to and possibly reliant on Roxanne's aura of competence and invulnerability. The group leaders praised her disclosure of this powerful experience to the rest of the group and validated her feelings of loss. They asked if any of the other group members had any thoughts or feelings about Roxanne's disclosure. No one spoke. In retrospect, even though Roxanne had a profound experience, the group leaders may have missed opportunities to help her explore her thoughts and emotions further. She continued to be a pleasant and cooperative group member but never discussed anything as personal again.

ALLISON: THE DEFENSIVE AND CONTROLLING GROUP MEMBER

Occasionally the need to maintain the appearance of having total control over the breast cancer experience and other life stressors is a sign of deep-seated personality traits. When these characteristics are revealed during stress management and relaxation training group interventions, group leaders must decide to what extent they should challenge the group member's defenses. One such participant, Allison, was a tremendous challenge to her group leaders.

Allison was a woman in her early 50s. She had a doctoral degree and was a research scientist with extensive knowledge of brain function, physiology, and neurology. Her expertise established her as the B-SMART group's authority on the human brain—a position normally reserved for the group leaders. She was very comfortable addressing issues scientifically and frequently directed the conversation back to her area of expertise. She described her method of coping with stress (breast cancer stress and other stress) as follows: "Gather all of the information you need, make your decisions, plan for the worst, and keep going." Although her approach seemed to overlap with some of the material presented in the intervention, one vital component was missing. Her approach left no room for emotion, emotion-focused coping, or softening. The group leaders soon discovered that inherent to Allison's "just do it" approach were distortions about her coworkers and other people in her life, a desire to prove that she did not need support, tremendous anger, a pervasive need to firmly control every aspect of her life, and a sense of isolation and loneliness.

When addressed by either of the group leaders, Allison would immediately become defensive. For example, in one session, Allison reported having been very upset when her teenage son came home very late one evening. One of the group leaders said that it sounded like she had felt worried and perhaps had been angry with him. She immediately minimized the amount of concern she had felt and went on to say, as she became more agitated, "It's just like a teenager to behave that way. They tell you one thing and then do something else. Their whole world is focused on themselves. He doesn't even acknowledge I have cancer." When the group leader again said that she seemed angry about the situation, Allison denied being upset. The group leader then shifted her approach and asked Allison to verbalize the thoughts she had in response to her son's lateness. She was either unable or unwilling to do so until some of the other group members started identifying them for her. Although she resisted being confronted by the group leaders, she seemed to accept a challenge from the other group members.

Throughout the intervention, Allison denied feeling any emotions about her cancer diagnosis and was unable and unwilling to work on identifying distortions in her own thinking. She was able to identify physiological changes associated with her stress (e.g., an increased heart rate, shortness of breath) but was unable to identify any subjective emotional experience associated with the physical changes. In Session 5, the group leaders decided to try to work more directly with Allison. Allison's defenses appeared to become fully activated. At one point, she said to one of the group leaders, "You want me to cry because I have breast cancer." The group leader responded, "Is that how it seems? Like I am trying to force you to cry?" Allison did not respond. The group leader continued, "I want to understand what the experience of having breast cancer is like for you." Allison then said, "Cancer has given me the opportunity to stop and appreciate everything in my life—to understand that the future is limited." This statement completely contradicted her reports that she had a lot of pressure in her life and was constantly rushing from one demand to the next. She started to cry. "What are you tears trying to say?" asked one of the group leaders. "That I am happy!" shouted Allison. "That every day is beautiful, and I am growing in my spirituality."

On the surface, Allison's words sounded right. Clinical supervision sessions became very intense as the group leaders tried to explore and explain the qualitative gap between Allison's words and the feeling in the room as Allison emphasized her well-being. The group leaders began to focus more intently on issues of countertransference. Simultaneously, they began to explore whether Allison's underlying schema, or personality structures, were contributing to the group leaders' difficulties with her. At the end of Session 7, the group leaders announced that the material for the next week would address anger. Allison became highly agitated, proclaiming anger served no good purpose and that as far as she was concerned, people should get rid of it as quickly as possible. One of the group leaders reflected back that Allison apparently had very strong feelings about anger and had a firmly entrenched working model for addressing anger. The group leader asked her to consider whether other models of anger might exist. She did not respond.

During Session 8, a group member who had not been present during Session 7 openly shared her experience of working through conflicting feelings about anger. She shared that she had been the victim of her father's anger throughout her abusive childhood. When she finished, she looked at Allison and said, "Now it's your turn." Visibly taken aback, Allison hesitated and then went on to reveal that she had also been abused as a child by her older sister and her mother. She reported that as a child, she felt weak because she was unable to control their rage toward her, regardless of what she did. As a result, she withdrew and became passive. She referred to her father as "a human vegetable" because of his inability and unwillingness to stop the mother and sister. She concluded by saying that this was the reason she felt anger had no purpose and wanted nothing to do with it. Later in the session, the group leaders acknowledged Allison's disclosure. They were able to use the information she offered to try and support her and help her realize that being passive as a child was a method of adapting to her family's uncontrollable and unpredictable anger.

Allison's disclosure allowed the group leaders a glimpse into her inner world. It was clear that even the smallest admission of vulnerability was frightening to Allison. They developed a strategy for the remaining sessions, which included fostering Allison's involvement with the other group members—they seemed to be developing lasting relationships, and Allison was responding with unbridled satisfaction. In addition, the group leaders decided to completely back away from challenging her or having her delve more deeply into her thoughts and feelings. It seemed quite possible that working with two female group leaders had activated a schema associated with her abusive female family members and was too much for Allison to tolerate.

Allison's example includes issues of countertransference. One of the group leaders initially felt inadequate when dealing with Allison and attributed those feelings to her own inexperience as a group leader, Allison's education, and Allison's scientific expertise. Later in the intervention, the other group leader, a psychologist with 20 years of experience, reported feeling generally uneasy and annoyed with Allison. The group leaders were reinforced by the supervision team for acknowledging their own issues and supported as they brought them to the supervisors' attention. The supervisors also challenged them to use those feelings to understand how Allison's world worked. For example, one group leader felt that nothing she could do would help her get through to Allison— the first indication that Allison had a tightly constructed and controlled inner world that did not allow for feelings of vulnerability. The leaders were also encouraged to depersonalize their interactions with Allison so that they could focus on how the intervention could benefit her most, given her history and limited ability to work with it at that time.

Working through countertransference in a CBSM group intervention is challenging. A CBSM session is not a "depth psychotherapy" group per se, in which participants expect to be confronted with their internal psychic structures. In addition, the sessions do not give members the opportunity to explore deep-seated personality characteristics to the extent normally needed for significant change. The B-SMART team considered the intervention a success for Allison because it helped her to establish friendships with women from her group. Given her isolated existence and alienated sense of self, opening herself up to group members' offers of friendship and her eventual reciprocity was significant for Allison, even though she may not have realized it.

During the last session, the other group members started spontaneously discussing how the program had benefited them. Allison rather brusquely stated, "It has helped me develop options for dealing with uncomfortable situations." The group leaders felt that the relaxation training visibly benefited Allison as well. During the first relaxation session, she was unable to take deep breaths. She said that she had never been able to do this because it made her feel like she was choking. Within three sessions, she reported that she was using deep breathing to help her "buy some space" during potentially stressful situations. By Session 7, she was able to take very deep breaths once she had reached a state of relaxation. One of the group leaders pointed this out to her in a later session, to which she replied, "Hmm."

MARTHA: THE OLDER, MORE SKEPTICAL PARTICIPANT

Frequently, participants begin stress management and relaxation training at the request of a loved one. People who do not actually think they are stressed (even though others in their life think stress is affecting them) often do one of two things. They either convince themselves that they do not need the help and drop out of the group (complaining driving in traffic to group each week is what is actually causing the stress), or they participate in the program but remain skeptical, perhaps throughout the intervention.

Martha was a 67-year-old housewife who strongly vocalized her uncertainty about the program at the pregroup assessment. She was so skeptical that she refused to sign one of the forms needed to process her involvement as a group member. During self-introductions in the first session, she stated that she was there because her husband wanted her to participate and because they both believed in contributing to scientific research. (Her participation occurred during the empirical validation stage of the B-SMART intervention.) She was withdrawn and appeared somewhat agitated throughout the first half of the session. When one of the group leaders asked for members to participate in the first exercise, Martha jumped in. She became animated and freely offered suggestions. During Session 2, when one of the group leaders was introducing the idea that emotions are adaptive and tell people something about their environments, Martha spontaneously said that she had recently been "experiencing overwhelming feelings of sadness and crying over nothing—just coming out of the blue." The group leader suggested that sadness implied a sense of loss and asked Martha to consider what she had lost. Martha immediately responded that she had lost both breasts when she chose a double mastectomy over a lumpectomy with chemotherapy. She continued, saying that she had never thought about mourning the loss of her breasts, but that was exactly what she was doing. After her disclosure, the group leaders remained quiet and let the feelings of loss settle over the room.

In our experience, it is rare for women at this stage of coping with the breast cancer experience to so quickly acknowledge the loss associated with breast cancer surgery. Our preferred approach for dealing with these feelings of loss is the same one we endorse for processing existential issues. When a participant brings up the issue and the feelings, we allow the individual and the other group members to "sit" with the emotion. By the second session, Martha, initially the skeptic, effectively led the group into dealing with feelings of loss. Some groups never get to this point. Throughout the 10-week intervention, Martha and the group leaders referred back to that session. Martha reported that she was no longer overcome by feelings of sadness and was not having any more crying spells. The group leaders later identified the session as an example of "softening" or "sitting with" a feeling and one that exemplified the adaptive functions of emotions.

Martha continued to be involved on every level. Sometimes she challenged and questioned the material as she struggled to understand its relevance in her life. During Session 5, she reported to the group that she had watched a psychologist on the *Oprah* talk show who used an approach similar to the B-SMART approach. She was particularly impressed because he had been talking about differentiating between controllable and uncontrollable aspects of stressful events. During Session 6, she reported that she had been pointing out the cognitive distortions of her *Oprah* book club friends and her husband. She acknowledged that she had been living according to the "shoulds" in her life. She gave an example of how she had identified and subsequently let go of some of the all-or-nothing thinking that had driven her perfectionist approach to her life. She identified the relaxation techniques that worked best for her and practiced them daily. She was the only group member who did all her homework and read ahead in her manual before each session.

At the end of the intervention, Martha spontaneously said, "This has helped me so much. I realize that all my life I have pressured myself and everyone else around me to always do everything perfectly. Now I feel like I can say, 'Does this really matter?' and let it go. But I don't understand why it took me so long to figure this out. Why don't we just intuitively know that this approach will be better for us?" One of the group leaders responded, "Let's look at what kind of cognitive distortion might be involved in that question. Is it possible that what you are really saying is that you *should* have been able to realize that this method of coping was better for you?" Martha responded that, yes, she had been using a "should" statement. The group leader pointed out that when people are born, they do not come into the world with a defined system for coping with stressors. They learn coping approaches. She then asked Martha, "Why do you think you should know how to do something without having had the opportunity to learn it before? You previously learned certain methods of coping, and now you have learned some new ones." Martha responded, "You're right. I didn't think I had to be a perfectionist when I was a baby or a little girl. Somewhere along the way, I learned to be a perfectionist. In fact, I learned it from my father. But now I can challenge that and replace the thoughts about everything needing to be perfect with, 'That will just have to be good enough. I'm doing the best I can given everything else I am dealing with.'"

FRANCESCA AND LOUISE: WORKING WITH DIFFERENT INTERPERSONAL STYLES

This two-person case study is interesting on many levels. One participant was a member of an ethnic minority, whereas the other was a member of the majority group represented in this particular group. Francesca and Louise were older than many of our participants and the other members of their own group. They were diametrically opposed in their levels of comfort with anger and their interpersonal styles.

Special Considerations for Ethnic Minority Participants

Francesca was a soft-spoken, withdrawn ethnic minority woman who initially revealed many symptoms of depression. She was very eager to participate in the intervention but was also very hesitant. She was the only member of her ethnic group in the B-SMART group. The other three members of the group were of the same ethnicity. One of the two group leaders was from yet another ethnic background. The three members with the same ethnicity seemed to begin to establish bonds early in the program, in spite of their age differences.

Francesca chose not to disclose very much information. When she did, it was almost inaudible. She was uncomfortable participating in group activities and avoided making eye contact. The group leaders were uncertain about how much to push her and did not know how much of her reticence was caused by her feeling uncomfortable about being the minority in the group and what other factors might be contributing to her reserved style. Because both of the group leaders were in training, group sessions were videotaped with the permission of the group members. Supervisors evaluating the session tapes noted that Francesca appeared depressed and feared that coming on too strongly might make her even more reluctant to participate.

Group leaders developed a strategy that involved matching Francesca's volume and tone of voice while warmly reaching out to her. Group leaders were encouraged to consistently but gently provide opportunities for her to participate. She slowly began to respond to overtures, would provide feedback during in-session exercises, and started to share her homework (which she completed religiously) when asked to do so. The fourth session was a breakthrough. During the relaxation exercise, Francesca was absolutely beaming. After the exercise ended, one of the group leaders commented on how happy and peaceful she looked while the relaxation script was being read. Francesca said that she had been transported to a place of such peace and beauty that she had not wanted to return back to the group. The group leaders reinforced her full engagement in the relaxation practice and encouraged her to share more about her experience. Louise also commented on how great Francesca seemed to have done with the relaxation. From that point on, Francesca started to open up and embrace the entire process. She worked on applying the stress management material to her own situation, even though it was extremely difficult to do so at times. In the session on anger (Session 8)—a subject with which Francesca was extremely uncomfortable—she shared some of her childhood experiences. In Session 9, she reported that she had spoken with a sibling about a childhood incident dating back almost 50 years that had never been addressed between them. She was amazed that her sibling did not remember the event, which had been so very significant for Francesca, but she was also very satisfied that she had been able to verbalize her pain after all of those years.

Indeed, Francesca seemed to find her voice during the 10-week intervention. The actual volume of her speech increased. She began to laugh out loud. You could see the depressive symptoms lifting from week to week. Had we assumed she was unwilling to participate and let her remain detached, she would never have made the marvelous breakthrough. Because she was a highly intelligent woman, she undoubtedly would have benefited from the program on many levels if we had allowed her to remain withdrawn, but it is unlikely that she would have blossomed the way she did.

Special Considerations for Older Women

The dynamics between older and younger group members should be assessed as quickly as possible. Often a warm, nurturing, and usually reciprocal relationship develops. Some younger and older members form mother–daughter relationships. They may connect and gain a sense of understanding that may not exist in the women's biological relationships because their mother or daughter does not have breast cancer. Unfortunately, this mother–daughter dynamic can become detrimental if the older participant assumes a mothering or self-sacrificing role and is unable to fulfill her own needs during the program. In other words, we have observed relationships between younger and older women wherein the older woman puts her own emotional needs on hold to care for the younger group member. Some older group members have even entered into this dynamic with younger group leaders, offering assistance and even bringing baked items for them. (Other older participants have commented about the youthfulness of some of our group leaders in what seemed to be an effort to establish some kind of age-related hierarchy.)

As mentioned, Francesca and Louise were both older than the other members of the group. They both tended to be more withdrawn when one or both of the younger members were present. When the younger members were not present, Francesca would talk about how she was concerned about them and felt they could benefit if they were present. It is essential that group leaders be aware of any tendency among group members to establish themselves as caretakers or to try to suggest that they do not need help or are less worthy of help, regardless of the unconscious reasons. We would never suggest that caring for others is in itself an unhealthy act. However, allowing this behavior to continue without understanding its intent, evaluating how it may interfere with the program's effectiveness, or staging an appropriate intervention may create a situation wherein the caretaker member (whether older or younger) avoids or is distracted from the internal focus needed to embrace and integrate the material. Group leaders may have to monitor their own actions to ensure they do not tacitly buy into a group member's caretaker role. The leaders may need to directly discuss the issue with these members.

Bringing Together Opposing Interpersonal Styles

Another wonderful event that transpired in this group was the connection that formed between Louise and Francesca. As mentioned, they were about the same age but were very different in almost every other respect. They were initially pleasant but somewhat distant with one another. As the intervention progressed, they began to openly discuss issues with one another. By the end of Session 7, they openly acknowledged the differences in their comfort levels with anger. Louise's childhood was filled with anger and abuse. She had learned to respond to even mildly provocative situations with anger. She was aware of this pattern and had worked on it in therapy several years previously. Even though it still seemed that she could be fairly easily provoked, she was a wonderful group member who eagerly discussed the material and rarely became defensive when the group leaders worked with her directly.

Francesca's background was somewhat less clear. According to Francesca, her childhood family home was typically characterized by high levels of anger, but actual expressions of this anger were not allowed. When anger was expressed, it was very powerful and frightening and accompanied by unpredictable behaviors. As a result, Francesca learned to fear anger and felt that it served no purpose. The group leaders spent significant time helping her understand that anger can be beneficial in that it can motivate people to act. It was very difficult for her to separate the emotion of anger from the violent and unpredictable behaviors she associated with it.

Louise shared examples of how she expressed her anger, and Francesca listened with a sense of awe. Louise's expressions of anger were sometimes aggressive or passive–aggressive. The only time Louise became somewhat defensive was when one of the group leaders pointed this out. During Session 8, the group leaders were faced with a formidable task— trying to move Louise and Francesca toward more moderate methods of anger expression when they were on opposite ends of the anger spectrum. The leaders decided to take a direct approach. The anger model presented involved two ways people typically handle anger: "stuffing" it (repressing it) or simply exploding. The group leader turned to Louise and Francesca and said, "This is kind of like the two of you. Louise, you say that you have always exploded, kind of like your dad used to. Francesca, you kind of hold your anger inside and let it eat at you." Francesca denied that she ever experienced anger. She emphasized that when someone upset her, she immediately forgave them. The leaders did not address the statement directly and continued with the lesson, pointing out that neither stuffing nor exploding is a healthy expression of anger because it does not allow people to communicate about the precipitating issues. Francesca and Louise grappled with the concept. Louise had a difficult time acknowledging that she was still a fairly angry, aggressive person. Francesca did not even want to talk about anger. The following week, Francesca discussed the confrontation with her sibling. Louise told the group that she had spoken directly with her boss about an incident. She told him that she had become angry when he used her as a scapegoat to deal with a difficult client. The group leaders heaped praise on both women. Francesca and Louise had both taken huge steps toward mitigating their stressful methods of managing anger. At one point during Session 9, Francesca turned to Louise and said, "I need more of what you've got." Louise replied, "And I need more of what you have." During the last session, the two exchanged telephone numbers and promised to stay in touch.

ASTRID: HANDLING DISEASE RECURRENCE OR METASTASIS

During Astrid's first group session, she recounted a horror story of oversights and mistakes by medical providers that she felt had led to her disease progression. She stated that her medical providers had ignored what she had considered to be obvious symptoms of cancer. Her story was marked with anxious and agitated statements and started to spin out of control. The other group members watched her with mounting tension until one of the group leaders gently stopped her, validated her stress, and redirected the group.

Astrid pulled herself together and from that point forward was fully engaged in the stress management material and relaxation training. She was progressing wonderfully and frequently set the tone for the group with her disclosures and bare-bones honesty about her cognitions, emotions, struggles, and successes with the material and other events in her life. In essence, she was a great group member. During Session 4, she announced that her doctors had found a tumor in the right frontal lobe region of her brain. The group members were initially stunned into silence. The group leaders, without saying a word, decided to let the group decide how far to go in their exploration of the issue. When it appeared that Astrid and the group were finished, the leaders offered Astrid support and tried to direct the remainder of the discussion back to the original session material. A significant chunk of the session had been spent processing this development, so much of the material had to be covered in the next session. After the session, the group leaders discussed how the news of Astrid's tumor might affect the group. The group leaders were prepared to help the group fully explore any existential issues that arose. They were also aware that they might have to skip some of the informational material to meet Astrid's and the group's needs.

We are including this case study so that potential group leaders will think through how they might handle a similar situation. Patients who are diagnosed in the later stages of breast cancer are more likely to develop metastases, have a recurrence, or develop new primary tumors. Although this intervention was originally designed for patients with early- to mid-stage breast cancer, it contains material that may be helpful in situations such as Astrid's. The second session on coping introduces emotion-focused coping and softening, which could be beneficial for a group member in this situation and for her fellow group members.

Be aware that group members may not want to process their responses to another group member's metastases or recurrence. Although most members will be concerned about and feel compassion for their fellow group member, it is likely that they will become worried about their own chances for recurrence. Ideally, a group would use two or three sessions to get past their initial shock and immediate fear response. They would be caring and empathetic toward the affected group member and then try to discuss the experience in the context of the coping lesson (e.g., controllable vs. uncontrollable aspects, problem-focused vs. emotion-focused coping). However, balancing the needs of the affected group member and their own fear responses may be far too overwhelming to quickly and neatly fit into the program's coping model. Given that most participants are just learning this type of approach to stress management, this scenario would be understandable. Group leaders must carefully determine how deeply they should explore the emotions involved in this type of situation, particularly if the situation occurs during the last weeks of the intervention (because members will have little time to process the emotional response). Our rule of thumb is, "Follow the group to the level they can tolerate." We let them show us the level of existential processing they are ready for and then gently probe a bit further. If we are repeatedly diverted away from the intensity of the issues at hand, we back off, understanding that the material may come up in discussions in later sessions.

Other Challenges for
Group Leaders

EXISTENTIAL ISSUES

How do group leaders know when to put the didactic material aside and address existential or other important topics that arise? Frankly, this is a difficult issue and one that we repeatedly address. More than anything, this decision involves clinical judgment. When one or both of the group leaders sense that an issue is not going to disappear (or conversely, that everyone would rather avoid it), try to encourage some processing. Often the issue at hand can be tied into previous or future lessons. When it ties into a future lesson, group leaders may defer the conversation and tell the group that it will be addressed specifically in a future session. Group leaders must be very careful to actually revisit the issue when the relevant session rolls around. If the material can be tied into previous material, do so. An effective technique is to ask other group members a question such as, "How might lessons from a few weeks ago address this issue?" Any suggestions offered are reinforced as good integration of the material. If none of them hit the mark, a group leader can say, "Yes, that seems to fit [or not], but I was actually thinking about. . . ." Group leaders should not be concerned about occasionally digressing from the scripted material to gain better understanding about individual or group processes or to address a pressing issue. However, every effort should be made to return to the material and reinforce its applicability to a wide variety of situations.

GROUP LEADERS' ANXIETIES ABOUT CANCER

Frequently, female group leaders become very anxious when beginning to work with breast cancer patients. One of our group leaders developed a muscle spasm over her left breast when she first joined our team. After judiciously having a breast examination, mammogram, and ultrasound to rule out the possibility of breast cancer, she acknowledged that she was having a somatic response to the anxiety generated by confronting the reality of breast cancer for the first time. After acknowledging the fear associated with the possibility of having breast cancer, the leader was able to reframe her thoughts about the disease and its treatment and to minimize her distress. After the first few sessions, another group leader who was experienced but new to the B-SMART project said that she felt uncomfortable being so involved in the experience of breast cancer in a group setting. She was surprised that she was feeling so uncomfortable but acknowledged her feelings and worked through them.

Each group leader has different vulnerability triggers that may be activated, even though the leaders are unaware of their existence. Younger team members have reported feeling vulnerable as younger group members share their experiences. It appears that age similarities often force group leaders to confront the possibility that they could develop breast cancer. Other factors that may trigger feelings of vulnerability during the intervention are breast tenderness (which is often a normal part of the menstrual cycle), a life history that is similar to a group member's, a family history of breast cancer, and problems with their breasts (e.g., cysts, other breast health issues). Undoubtedly, other factors exist as well. Just hearing the stories of women who are receiving treatment for breast cancer and are in the midst of a disease-related crisis can cause group leaders to become anxious. This is a normal and adaptive response because it can motivate them to maintain a regular examination schedule.

As group leaders continue to work with patients with breast cancer, having an inside glimpse of their resilience becomes a source of strength. The women we work with are remarkable in their determination to beat the disease and continue their lives—hopefully, less stressfully. In addition, group leaders learn firsthand that people can survive the disease—now more than ever . With early detection and treatment, most women survive breast cancer and resume normal lives within a relatively short period.

The information in this paragraph is provided for group leaders who are attempting to manage the personal stress associated with working among cancer patients. We do not normally discuss the specifics of treatment-related developments with our group members—they usually do this among themselves. We think that group members can best cope with these developments by relying on each other. Regardless, group leaders may develop some significant concerns about the members as they move through the 10 weeks of the program. Concerns about breast cancer surgeries are best addressed by acknowledging that the loss of a body part is a painful but survivable experience, physically and emotionally. Adjuvant treatments, although certainly unpleasant, are also survivable and much more tolerable than they have been in the past. The side effects of chemotherapy that normally concern people the most are gastrointestinal symptoms and hair loss. Both effects of the treatment are temporary. Many medications can be used to mitigate vomiting and nausea, and hair grows back very quickly after treatment cessation. In other words, hair loss is also temporary and survivable. In addition, exploring the possible distortions involved in anticipating the negative effects of chemotherapy is a tough but powerful way to emphasize the salience of the B-SMART intervention.

One group leader discovered a palpable mass in her breast during the eighth week of the 10-week intervention. Undoubtedly, her heightened awareness of the disease was the result of her relatively long-term involvement with the project. This awareness and her subsequent concern motivated her to move as quickly as possible. When she tried to make an appointment with a specialist, she was told the next available appointment was approximately 6 weeks away. The thought of living with the uncertainty for that amount of time felt like it would be more stressful than finding out she had cancer and starting to cope with the disease. She called her internist for help and was seen by a specialist within 24 hours. The specialist performed an aspiration of the mass, and then she found out that she had to wait for at least 4 days to get the results. When she went to work, she used many of the program's coping and relaxation techniques. Regardless, she freely admits that those 4 days were tremendously stressful. She felt that she no resolution of her questions and concerns and was unable to plan her next course of action. She was amazed at the powerful sense of relief that washed over her when she received the news that the mass was not cancerous. She readily acknowledged that she was stressed during the 4 days, yet she had no idea how intense her feelings were until the situation was resolved and she was flooded with relief.

This experience and her ability to articulate its various components gave this group leader insight into the early stages of the stress and coping responses. Our participants have navigated through several of the most stressful aspects of the cancer experience by the time they begin our intervention. Thus, we rarely hear about the 6- to 8-week waiting periods preceding the definitive diagnosis and the stress associated with waiting for a diagnosis. Nor do we hear about the anticipatory stress associated with a surgery. Most participants who are just beginning the B-SMART intervention are distressed about chemotherapy or radiation treatment. The importance of the revelations gained from this group leader's experience is the understanding that our participants have been living with uncertainty, anticipation, and stress for approximately 2 to 3 months before they even begin the B-SMART program. We wonder how our program could benefit women if we began working with them earlier in the process. We sincerely hope others will evaluate the merits of using this program for women who have just received their diagnosis.

The other salient issue from the group leader's experience once again involves group leaders' responses to working with women who have cancer. This particular group leader was able to conduct the final session of her group. Still, before she learned that the mass was benign, she found it difficult to sit through the supervision sessions and even the team research meetings. She said that listening to the clinical discussions about group members' experiences angered and frightened her. She had not told the team about her situation and did not want to do so during a supervision or research session. When team members began speculating about a given group member, she wished that she could forcefully explain, "You just don't understand how *frightening* the experience is even when you have a fairly extensive coping arsenal at your disposal!" She reports now that she has tried to use her experience to make her more empathetic toward the participants. She recognizes that she has not experienced what it feels like to have breast cancer and undergo the treatments, but she has gotten a glimpse of how upsetting it can be. She says that her own foray into the world of breast disease has increased her respect for the resiliency of the women who have participated in the B-SMART program.

Assessing Progress in the B-SMART Program | 5

What Is the Purpose of Assessment in Clinical Validation of Psychosocial Interventions?

How does one screen for participants who might benefit most from the B-SMART intervention? How does one monitor progress in the B-SMART intervention program? In many ways, our approach to these questions was guided by a 1995 report from a task force assembled by the American Psychological Association (APA). The *APA Task Force on Psychological Intervention Guidelines* outlined several methods for ensuring the validity of psychosocial interventions for mental disorders and psychosocial aspects of physical disorders (APA, 1995). The task force stated that any evaluation of an intervention program should provide a cumulative database of assessments allowing for a systematic review of experimental replications through sophisticated techniques such as meta-analysis. The large sample resulting from a history of replication studies also allows one to address the issue of matching patients and treatments. In other words, which individual-differences variables (e.g., personality, demographic, medical) predict an optimal response to a given intervention? This question about the assessment process can be answered during screening. Not only can patients' characteristics be used to predict optimal treatment responses at this time, but screening interviews can also be used to identify patients who have more severe psychiatric issues (e.g., are severely depressed or suicidal). These patients may be less appropriate for group-based CBSM intervention and may benefit more from an intensive individual psychotherapy or pharmacological intervention. It follows that the assessment battery chosen involves factors addressing patient/treatment matching issues as well as those traditionally used for evaluating the efficacy of an intervention. Although the former often involves stable traits or characteristics or severe psychopathological conditions, the latter must include measures that are sensitive to change in functioning over time (i.e., pre–post treatment and follow-up).

The APA report noted that "all interventions should be subject to empirical confirmation," and "each intervention should be subjected to an increasingly stringent set of methodologies designed to enhance confidence in the efficacy of that intervention" (pp. 8–9). The report further noted that randomized controlled clinical trials are one of the most stringent means of evaluating treatment efficacy and can be used to determine whether the treatment is better than no treatment, whether the intervention is superior to others that contain factors common to all treatments, and how the treatment compares with other alternative interventions (e.g., pharmacological).

The APA Task Force report states specifically that outcome measures defining the effectiveness of an intervention should assess appropriate dimensions of the psychological state and disorder being addressed by the intervention; include measures of life functioning that encompass social and occupational functioning, relationship status, and subjective well-being; and address patient satisfaction. They also state that this assessment process should include outcomes that specify actual clinical benefits of the intervention (e.g., physical health changes, indicators of a normalization of functioning). Additional functions of the assessment battery include the following:

- Measures of the "dose of treatment" (e.g., number of sessions attended, patient adherence to intervention guidelines, frequency of out-of-session use of intervention techniques)
- Manipulation checks to document whether the intervention had its specific intended effects on proximal intervention targets (e.g., whether a person's distorted cognitive appraisals actually changed during the course of a cognitive–behavioral therapy program)
- Identification of patient variables (e.g., cultural background, gender, age, socioeconomic status, personality characteristics, physical condition) that may moderate the effects of the intervention (a requirement that relates to the issue of preintervention screening and baseline assessment)

What Is the Purpose of Assessment in Clinical Treatment?

This chapter addresses ways to approach the B-SMART program assessment process—specifically, how to collect data at each of these levels. Some clinicians may be particularly interested in screening measures, whereas others may be more focused on conducting regular manipulation checks or collecting repeated measurements of outcome variables.

Although many of these assessment goals and strategies are critical for establishing treatment efficacy, practitioners planning to use the B-SMART program are much more likely to be concerned with a minimal number of screening issues, indicators of treatment effectiveness (e.g., single measures of distress reduction and daily functioning), actual clinical changes, and other data that pertain to the issues of generalizability of the intervention to different patients, feasibility of the intervention across patients and settings, and the costs and benefits associated with administering the intervention (APA, 1995).

We have used interviews, questionnaires, and bioassays to assess variables in each of these domains throughout the research and development phase of the B-SMART program. Specifically, the assessments most pertinent to establishing the efficacy of the program are the assessments that document the following:

- Patient characteristics (to address demographic, personality, and contextual factors that may assist with patient/treatment matching and treatment generalizability issues)
- Patient adherence (to address treatment dose and patient involvement)
- Manipulation checks (to address skill acquisition and retention)
- Treatment outcomes (to address treatment efficacy)

This chapter presents the assessment strategies we used during the development and evaluation of the B-SMART program so that it can be used as a model by others who are interested in developing psychosocial intervention programs for addressing other behavioral medicine issues in people with breast cancer or other diseases. By providing suggestions for abbreviated assessment batteries, we address the needs of clinicians who will be implementing the B-SMART intervention in a multidisciplinary service environment. Finally, the chapter includes a discussion of the ways in which a systematic evaluation of the B-SMART program could be implemented at multiple treatment sites so that we can continue to build a database supporting the effectiveness of the program and to use to address issues of patient/treatment matching and generalizability.

Assessment of Patient Characteristics at Screening

From the standpoint of clinical practice, it is important to keep in mind that the B-SMART intervention is not a panacea for all of the mental health issues that women with breast cancer may have. As mentioned previously, some women may have such overwhelming depressive symptoms that they are unable to commit to a 10-week program or even focus on the group sessions. These women may be best served by an initial round of intensive individual psychotherapy or a pharmacological regimen that allows them to manage their symptoms. Perhaps then they would be excellent candidates for the B-SMART program. In other words, the initial screening battery should assess the presence of severe psychopathological symptoms. It may also be used to measure other more subtle indicators of psychological status, as well as physical functioning and medical treatment status, to help determine when a woman is ready to begin the B-SMART program. A woman who has only been recovering from surgery for a few days would not be ready to assimilate the information discussed in the B-SMART sessions.

The screening process may be equally important in a research setting or program evaluation. When attempting to validate the effectiveness of a specific intervention, it is important in the preliminary stages to obtain a sample that is as homogeneous as possible to reduce the likelihood that extraneous variables are affecting the measurements of the intervention. Including a set of inclusion and exclusion criteria that are enforced throughout the initial efficacy trials can help ensure this type of homogeneity. Extraneous variables can have a substantial impact on the process or outcome of some psychosocial interventions, variables that include psychiatric disorders, psychopharmacological regimens that have just begun, disease progression, serious side effects of adjuvant therapy, and other ongoing physical symptoms associated with sleep loss and fatigue. In a research setting the influence of these external factors can be controlled by using a stringent set of inclusion and exclusion criteria, although sometimes the use of exclusion as a control method is simply not feasible. Suspected extraneous variables that are either highly prevalent in the target population (e.g., alcohol use, sleep disruptions, use of aerobic exercise) or make up the demographic characteristics of the target population (e.g., age, ethnicity, socioeconomic status) can be controlled by repeated (i.e., preintervention and postintervention) assessments of "control variables" for inclusion as covariates in statistical analyses. Finally, as one moves past efficacy trials and more closer toward effectiveness trials, the necessity of incorporating a more heterogeneous sample (i.e., real-world people with cancer) means that not all of these criteria will be able to be controlled by selection.

COLLECTING INFORMATION

To collect a comprehensive set of assessments in a standardized way, we have developed a suggested screening battery that progressively probes for inclusion and exclusion criteria. The first tier of this battery includes phone screening to detect the presence of gross psychopathology (based on self-reported hospital admissions, ongoing psychiatric medications, or self-reported substance abuse or dependency and symptoms of major depressive disorder) or women with advanced stages of breast cancer (based on diagnostic tests or examinations). We determined that the presence of gross psychopathology or advanced breast cancer could be serious confounders and might limit participants' ability to benefit from the intervention.

A second tier in the assessment process involves psychiatric interviews and questionnaires to detect the severity of more subtle signs and symptoms of psychopathology or to detect factors that may preclude an individual's benefiting from or contributing to an intervention group. At this stage of the screening process, we use the 17-item Hamilton Rating Scale for Depression (HRS-D; Hamilton, 1960) and the Hamilton Rating Scale for Anxiety (HRS–A; Hamilton, 1959). The Structured Clinical Interview for *DSM–IV* (SCID; First, Spitzer, Gibbons, & Williams, 1995) may be used to detect the presence of Axis I clinical disorders including but not limited to affective disorders such major depressive episode, acute anxiety disorders, thought disorders, and substance dependency. The SCID assesses current and lifetime psychotic disorders and disorders of mood, psychoactive substance use, anxiety, and *DSM–IV* adjustment disorders.

To detect the presence of Axis II personality disorders, we use of a two-step process that includes an abbreviated interview to detect issues uncovered by the administration of the SCID–II (Spitzer, Williams, Gibbon, & First, 1990). Such issues include a tendency to monopolize conversations, have difficulty maintaining boundaries, and demonstrate wide variations in emotions. One can administer the SCID–II to screen specifically for personality disorders, such as antisocial personality disorder and borderline personality disorder, that could be particularly disruptive to a group-based psychosocial intervention. It is highly likely that individuals with these disorders would find it difficult to benefit from a group intervention and would be disruptive in the group (Ironson, Antoni, &

Lutgendorf, 2002). The main assessment mission at this point in the screening process is to establish whether a potential participant would be an appropriate group member. As noted by Ironson et al. (2002), appropriate individuals should be able to listen to conversations, share their experiences openly, be willing to participate in group discussions, and cooperate by completing several short exercises and mini-assessments that are used in the intervention. As mentioned previously, less appropriate individuals include those who monopolize conversations, are extremely uncomfortable with or unwilling to speak in a group, lack the energy or motivation to participate, are having psychotic thoughts or showing psychotic behaviors, tend to have impulsive or otherwise inappropriate anger responses (which could divide group members), have difficulty with boundaries (e.g., make inappropriate advances toward the interviewer), or are struggling with a substance dependency or other life circumstance that precludes their ability to attend regular meetings, assimilate information, and complete out-of-session activities (e.g., relaxation practice and self-monitoring).

Note that the SCID and SCID–II are designed to aid in the diagnosis of disorders that meet *DSM–IV* criteria for a mental health condition. As such, each instrument is focused on a level of psychopathology that might be observed in psychiatric populations. It is possible that the SCID may not be as sensitive to more subtle levels of mood changes (e.g., depressed affect), or the SCID–II may not be sensitive to the more subtle variations in personality style that capture some of the tendencies just noted. During the assessment for the presence of these characteristics, it may be helpful to use a measure that taps the full range of mood-related states and personality style characteristics and has been designed specifically for patients dealing with nonpsychiatric medical conditions. One such instrument is the Millon Behavioral Medicine Diagnostic (MBMD; Millon, Antoni, Millon, Meagher, & Grossman, 2001). The MBMD provides information that may be quite relevant during screening, such as information on the full range of mood states related to Axis I, 11 personality styles that reflect milder degrees of tendencies reflected in Axis II, and a wide collection of scales assessing stress-moderating resources (e.g., social support, spirituality), illness perceptions, health habits, and issues related to treatment (e.g., tendencies toward medication abuse, noncompliance, overuse of services).

Clinicians deciding to implement some of these screening procedures may want to abbreviate the assessment process by using other interviews, fewer modules of the SCID, or shorter self-report instruments such as the MBMD. Given the prevalence of certain issues in patients with breast cancer, the SCID modules that may be the most useful include those on affective disorders, anxiety disorders, psychotic disorders, psychoactive substance use disorders, and adjustment disorders. Although the first four of these modules may provide reasonable grounds for excluding a person from a stress management group, we have found that individuals diagnosed with adjustment disorders are very commonly encountered in clinical practice, and they may be able to benefit greatly from a program such as B-SMART.

Physical and laboratory test criteria used in the B-SMART validation studies were designed to create homogeneous samples of study participants so that we could (a) minimize the contribution of extraneous variables (e.g., differences in disease stage) to outcome measures and (b) ensure that the topics and their resulting discussions would be equally pertinent to all group members.

The latter goal is likely to be important to clinicians using this intervention because groups composed of individuals at different disease stages (i.e., groups with a mix of patients who have early-stage disease and those who have metastatic disease and overt symptoms) may be upsetting for some group members. In addition, a mixed group may raise so many additional topics during discussions that the intervention becomes less effective. On the other hand, individuals with early-stage disease may learn a lot from these sorts of discussions (e.g., it may decrease their sense of uncertainty about the future of their disease course), so some groups may be better served by greater disease stage heterogeneity. Decisions concerning the criteria to be used for forming these groups are ultimately made by the clinician conducting the B-SMART intervention.

SPECIAL ISSUES: SUICIDAL TENDENCIES AND EXTREME DISTRESS REACTIONS

During the course of phone interviews and face-to-face interviews with women who have been recently diagnosed with and treated for breast cancer and who are being considered for the B-SMART program, it is possible to encounter individuals who reveal that they have attempted suicide, either quite recently or in the distant past. In a situation like this, it is important for the person conducting the assessment to assess the individual's current risk for suicide by collecting information on previous attempts, details of any recent attempts (i.e., in the past few weeks), recurrent suicidal ideation or intentions, and whether the person has a suicide plan (and if so, whether the plan is detailed). If an interviewer decides that an individual is currently at risk for committing suicide, the interviewer needs to refer the person to a psychiatric facility for immediate care. If a person mentions suicidal ideation during the course of a screening interview but does not have a specific plan, please be aware that other factors may increase the person's risk of suicide. Such factors include a history of previous suicide attempts with a high lethality, possessing the means to commit suicide, substance abuse or dependence, a history of mood disorders or other psychiatric disorders, health problems, social isolation, multiple life stressors, and relationship problems. Special attention should be paid to any mention of suicidal ideation or intent during the initial screening interviews. Although individuals who are actively suicidal or having serious suicidal ideation would not be good candidates for the B-SMART program, they can be recontacted after they have received acute care and become stabilized.

The clinician should also be prepared to either treat or refer for treatment individuals who are unable to qualify for the B-SMART program because of other mental health problems including acute anxiety disorders (e.g., panic attacks), psychotic disorders, and substance use disorders (e.g., alcohol or psychoactive substance abuse and dependency). Some of these individuals may benefit from a more structured, individually tailored supportive intervention.

Assessment of Participant Adherence and Treatment Dose

ATTENDANCE AT INTERVENTION SESSIONS

Group leaders may decide to record the frequency of attendance at each B-SMART session to assess the relationship between treatment dose and effectiveness. We have recorded attendance rates ranging from 60% to 100% in the 10-week CBSM-based interventions for participants with a wide variety of medical diseases. Attendance rates for the B-SMART intervention in our validation studies have been nearly 90%. We have also noted in some groups that better attendance is associated with greater benefits from the program (Ironson et al., 1994).

OUT-OF-SESSION ADHERENCE

To assess treatment adherence, we require participants in the B-SMART group to maintain daily self-monitoring records of relaxation practice frequency and perceived stress (see *Participant's Workbook*). Participants complete the equivalent of daily self-monitoring cards or sheets, indicating the total number of self-reported relaxation sessions practiced that day and recording a subjective rating of their distress level just before and just after the exercise. We have used these figures to compute the total frequency of relaxation practice sessions during the 10 weeks of the program (the total dose) and the total number of weeks in which participants practiced relaxation at least once at home (consistency). Lutgendorf et al. (1997) found that during the 10 weeks of a CBSM program, the average frequency of relaxation practice sessions by men with HIV infection was 4 times a week, with weekly averages varying from 0 to 14 sessions of relaxation. These averages are very similar to those reported in our previous work involving asymptomatic men participating in the CBSM program while they were being tested for HIV infection (Antoni et al., 1991). This study found that a greater frequency of relaxation home practice sessions during the 5 weeks preceding HIV antibody testing and notification was associated with lower depression and anxiety levels in the week after notification of HIV antibody test results (Antoni et al., 1991). Ironson and colleagues (1994) studied the same asymptomatic men and found that greater relaxation practice frequency was significantly associated with less disease progression to AIDS ($r = -.71$, $p < .05$) 2 years later.

In a more recent study of men with HIV and HIV symptoms, it was found that consistency of relaxation practice sessions affects mood change more than the actual number of relaxation sessions that are practiced during the 10-week program (Lutgendorf et al., 1997). Specifically, we found that although the total number of relaxation practice sessions was not significantly associated with changes in depression and anxiety during the 10-week intervention program, the number of weeks that an individual practiced relaxation at least once was significantly correlated with changes in depression ($r = -.53$, $p = .02$) and anxiety ($r = -.51$, $p = .03$). In a later study (S. Cruess, Antoni, Cruess, et al., 2000), we found that greater reductions in stress levels after home practice of relaxation exercises related to greater improvements in immune status (i.e., decrements in antibody titers to genital herpes virus [HSV-2]). Thus, it appears that regularity of relaxation practice—and the stress reduction achieved during home relaxation practice—rather than the total number of relaxation sessions is associated with greater reductions in depression and anxiety and changes in immune status.

COMPLETION OF TAKE-HOME ACTIVITIES

We also assess participants' take-home assignments for adherence to various stress management aspects of the B-SMART protocol. All of these assessment materials are included in the *Participant's Workbook*. Typically these assignments ask participants to list the various stressful situations they encounter during the week and then use the stress management techniques discussed that week (e.g., cognitive restructuring, coping skills training, anger management, assertiveness training) to begin modifying their distress. Assessing adherence to these assignments is critical in determining the extent to which participants are using the skills learned during group sessions in their daily lives. Clinicians can assess adherence by asking to see the work done by participants, determining the number of stressful situations that are listed and analyzed, and checking the accuracy of the work completed. For example, one way to assess adherence to cognitive restructuring homework assignments is to count the number of negative thoughts that participants have attempted to restructure. This simple quantitative assessment allows the clinician to review the participant's level of motivation and willingness to comply with the protocol. In addition, clinicians should assess the accuracy of participants' labeling of cognitive distortions and their ability to generate rational thought replacements that parallel reductions in negative mood reports. Clinicians may want to pay special attention to participants' performance on assignments during Sessions 3 through 5 of the program to ensure that they have developed the basic cognitive restructuring skills necessary to benefit from the techniques taught in subsequent sessions (i.e., coping skills, anger management, assertiveness). Problems in these assignments (e.g., too few assignments completed, inaccurate application of stress management strategies) can be addressed during the group session and subsequently corrected.

Of course, clinicians continue this quantitative and qualitative assessment of take-home assignments throughout the 10-week protocol, which allows them to determine the extent to which participants have assimilated relevant material from each session. Homework assignments should be assessed at the beginning of each group session. If participants realize that their assignments will be analyzed and discussed during the session, it is likely to improve their compliance. Maintaining a weekly record of quantitative and qualitative adherence rates allows clinicians to notice improvements made by group members and reinforce their achievements. Such reinforcement is likely to motivate them to continue completing these assignments diligently during the 10-week protocol and maintain their efforts after completion of the stress management program.

Assessment of Skill Acquisition and Treatment Mastery: Manipulation Checks

The various assessment methods for monitoring participants' retention of each of the major treatment components in the B-SMART program are summarized in Table 5.1, as are the major goals of the program. Monitoring the progress of participants as they progress through the 10 weeks

TABLE 5.1

Aims, Strategies, and Retention Measures for the B-SMART Program

Aims	Strategies	Retention measures
Increase awareness of stress responses and related processes.	Provision of information, provision of in-session experiences	In-session self-reports of awareness levels
Teach anxiety reduction skills.	PMR, imagery tapes, self-monitoring	PMR practice frequency, in-session behavioral observation[a]
Modify cognitive appraisals.	Cognitive restructuring	Homework assignments[b] in *Participant's Workbook* (Sessions 3 to 5)
Build coping skills and increase emotional expressiveness.	Assertion training, anger management	Homework assignments[b] skills and emotional expression in *Participant's Workbook* (Sessions 8 and 9)
Reduce social isolation.	Group support, social network enhancement strategies	In-session awareness exercise in *Participant's Workbook* (Session 7)

[a]Behavioral observation of muscle tension, posture, and breathing (Luiselli et al., 1979).
[b]Homework performance can be coded as the percentage of *Participant's Workbook* assignments completed.

of the program is a key responsibility of the clinician running this program because the relaxation and stress management techniques proceed from simple building blocks (e.g., awareness of cognitive appraisals about stressors) to more advanced combinations (e.g., changing distorted cognitive appraisals about social support resources before using assertive communication to elicit more support). Once a clinician becomes aware that a participant is stuck or cannot fully grasp a technique, the clinician should allow the participant to participate in extra in-session exercises (e.g., role-playing assertive communication) or provide additional out-of-session assignments.

AWARENESS OF STRESS RESPONSE PROCESSES

We have developed several in-session exercises and out-of-session homework activities to help participants increase their awareness levels of several subtle stress-related processes, including *signs of stress responses* (in cognitive, emotional, behavioral, physical, and social domains), *cognitive appraisals* (including appropriate and distorted thinking patterns), *coping strategies* (including direct and indirect problem- and emotion-focused strategies), *anger responses* (including a range of explosive anger responses and suppressed anger responses), *communication style* (passive, aggressive, passive–aggressive, and assertive), and *social resources* (social supports for emotional and instrumental purposes). Participants' performance in any of these domains can be used to judge their improvements in awareness levels. This step is critical because one premise of the B-SMART program is that individuals have to become *aware* of the characteristics and inefficiencies of their stress response processes before they can change them.

RELAXATION SKILLS

To assess acquisition of progressive muscle relaxation (PMR) skills, we use a behavioral observation protocol (Luiselli, Marholin, & Steinman, 1979) conducted by one of the two group leaders during the relaxation induction in each weekly session. This procedure allows the leaders to assess visually apparent muscle tension, breathing, and other physical changes during the relaxation session and then to score these changes from 1 to 10 on a 10-point scale. A leader can conduct this observation protocol during each of the 10 weekly B-SMART sessions to assess whether participants are improving their skills overall or are having difficulty relaxing any muscle groups. A few participants have reported that focusing on the tension levels in their arm muscles is anxiety arousing because it reminds them of how much muscle they have lost or of pain from lymphadema as a result of adjuvant therapy. In these cases, we have recommended that the participants focus exclusively on the sense of relaxation that they experience when they engage in the "relax" portion of the PMR exercise. Clinicians who would like to use this behavioral observation system should be aware that either two group leaders must be present (one to record the relaxation ratings while the other reads aloud the relaxation or imagery script) or the session will have to be videotaped and rated later. We have found that some women who have undergone radiation therapy or are experiencing hot flashes as side effects from hormonal treatments such as tamoxifen may feel physically uncomfortable during autogenics exercises involving suggestions of warmth or during relaxation imagery exercises that involve sunlight or heat. These women can be provided with alternative autogenic suggestions of heaviness instead of heat or alternative images that focus on color instead of sunlight. Clinicians using the B-SMART program should have these alternative scripts available.

COGNITIVE RESTRUCTURING SKILLS

Cognitive restructuring skills are assessed by participants' performance on take-home assignments designed to teach rational thought replacement in stressful circumstances. These assignments begin during Session 3 at a very basic level. Participants are required to record their weekly stressful events and the automatic thoughts (self-talk), feelings, and stress-associated physical symptoms associated with the events. Participants complete progressively more detailed assignments during the next 2 weeks. The cognitive restructuring assignments culminate in the completion of a five-step rational thought replacement assignment in which they are asked to think of as many as three separate stressful interactions or events and do the following for each interaction: (a) identify irrational or distorted self-talk, (b) rate their degree of belief in each negative thought, (c) challenge or dispute the self-talk, (d) replace the negative self-talk with a more rational response, and (e) evaluate the outcome of this process by rating their degree of belief in the self-talk and the emotional changes they experienced during the rational thought replacement. Group leaders can observe each participant's progress in identifying, challenging, and changing cognitive distortions and address troublesome areas as needed.

WITHIN-SESSION MOOD CHANGES

We also assess participants' mood state at the beginning and end of each B-SMART session using an abbreviated form of the Profile of Mood States (POMS) called the Incredibly Short POMS (Dean, Whelan, & Meyers, 1989). The Incredibly Short POMS is a 6-item version of the 65-item POMS (McNair, Lorr, & Droppelman, 1981) that assesses tension and anxiety, depression, anger, fatigue, vigor, and confusion. In addition to providing a running check on participants' mood state within and across the 10 B-SMART sessions, this assessment also helps participants become more aware of subtle differences between their mood states.

Assessment of Treatment Outcome

The efficacy of the B-SMART program was ultimately tested with a large battery of psychosocial outcome measures of depressive symptoms, distress levels, and quality of life. In addition to these outcome measures, we have systematically assessed changes in psychological variables that— as the proximal intervention targets of the B-SMART program—have been hypothesized to mediate these primary psychosocial outcomes. As discussed in the following section, clinicians who would like to monitor changes in patients who are completing the B-SMART program may choose to use a more abbreviated battery of tests that can be administered in a questionnaire or an interview form.

PSYCHOSOCIAL OUTCOMES MEASURES

We chose the following instruments to assess the domains relevant to individuals coping with breast cancer. We developed certain measures to specifically address the concerns of patients with cancer, whereas others address more general distress levels.

Depressive Symptoms

Depression is assessed with the Beck Depression Inventory (BDI; Beck, Ward, Mendelson, Mock, & Erbaugh, 1961), a 21-item inventory frequently used to assess cognitive, affective, and vegetative symptoms of depression. The BDI is thought to be more useful for assessing the severity of a depressive syndrome than for diagnosing depression (Kendall, Hollon, Beck, Hammen, & Ingram, 1987). Alternatively, depression can be assessed with the Center for Epidemiological Studies Depression Scale (CES–D; Radloff, 1977). We have found this instrument to be particularly sensitive to mood changes among patients in the B-SMART program who have early-stage breast cancer (Antoni et al., 2001).

General Distress

A modified version of the POMS (McNair et al., 1981) was used to measure changes in overall distressed mood (Carver et al., 1993) that occurred by the end of the 10-week intervention (in contrast to the Incredibly Short POMS, which was used to monitor within-session changes). The POMS, a widely used scale, is composed of adjectives that participants rate according to their mood during the previous week. Several mood states are assessed: anxiety, depression, anger, vigor, fatigue, and confusion. Each of these is rated on a 5-point scale, with 0 indicating *not at all* and 4 indicating *extremely*. The negative subscales are added, and the vigor subscale is subtracted, resulting in a total mood disturbance score. We have found that the scores for subscales identifying anxiety, depression, anger, and total mood disturbance decrease significantly during CBSM intervention (Antoni et al., 1991; Antoni, Cruess, Cruess, et al., 2000; Lutgendorf et al., 1997). The POMS is a particularly good instrument for assessing distress in the program because it is brief and has frequently been used to assess distress changes during the course of time-limited psychosocial interventions in other populations dealing with cancer and its treatment (e.g., Fawzy, Cousins, et al., 1990).

Cancer-Specific Distress

Because depression may not be as severe in some people with breast cancer and because fluctuations in depressive symptoms during the intervention may not reflect the changes in adjustment specific to dealing with cancer, we have also monitored cancer-specific distress changes using the Impact of Event Scale (IES; Horowitz et al., 1979). The IES is a 15-item self-report measure designed to explore intrusive thoughts and avoidant cognitions related to a traumatic life event. We have tailored the IES to assess participants' reports of intrusive thoughts and avoidant cognitions that are specifically related to having breast cancer. This instrument, which measures recurring thoughts and rumination, was chosen because of the high probability that patients with breast cancer have substantial fears about disease progression (Spencer et al., 1999). The IES can be adjusted to focus on other concerns such as fears of dependency, grave illness, or death.

Quality of Life

Quality of life is an elusive construct and can be operationalized in many ways. We have monitored changes in different quality-of-life dimensions using selected psychosocial subscales of the Sickness Impact Profile (SIP; Bergner, Bobbitt, Carter, & Gilson, 1981) and the Health Status Questionnaire Short Form (SF–36; Ware & Sherbourne, 1992). The SIP psychosocial subscales that focus on social functioning (i.e., social interactions and recreational pastimes) may be useful for evaluating the effects of the B-SMART program. We have also used the SF–36 to assess several general quality-of-life issues related to health. The SF–36 is a 36-item instrument with eight multi-item scales: (a) physical functioning, (b) *social functioning*, (c) *role limitations* caused by physical health problems, (d) *role limitations* caused by personal or emotional problems, (e) *general mental health*, (f) *vitality*, (g) *bodily pain*, and (h) *general health perceptions*. Subscale reliabilities have ranged from .81 to .88 among a large community-based sample of adults (Stewart et al., 1989; Stewart, Hays, & Ware, 1988). The SF–36 also has been used to evaluate functional status in individuals who are depressed, individuals who are chronically ill, and healthy individuals (Wells et al., 1989). The SF–36 has been tested in more than 60 populations and appears to provide a brief but comprehensive measure of functional status. To assess cancer-specific quality-of-life issues, clinicians can use the version of the Functional Assessment of

Cancer Therapy (FACT; Cella, Tulsky, et al., 1993) corresponding to the cancer that is the focus of the intervention. For example, the FACT-B would be used for patients with breast cancer. These relatively brief indexes can provide clinicians with a quick assessment of the areas that may be of particular importance to participants during the intervention program.

Fatigue

We use two scales to measure fatigue symptomatology: the Fatigue Symptom Inventory (FSI; Hann et al., 1998) and the Multidimensional Fatigue Symptom Inventory–Short Form (MFSI–SF; K. Stein, Martin, Hann, & Jacobsen, 1998). The FSI is a 14-item self-report measure that is designed to measure the intensity and frequency of fatigue and its impact on quality of life. All items (except those measuring number of days of fatigue—Items 12 and 13) are rated on 11-point scales (0 = *not at all fatigued*, 10 = *as fatigued as I could be*). Number of days ranges from 0 to 7 in the past week. Items 1 through 4 are added to provide an index of *fatigue intensity*. Items 5 through 11 are added to compute a *total disruption* index, and Items 12 and 13 yield a *fatigue frequency* score. The MFSI–SF is a 30-item self-report measure designed to measure the principal manifestations of fatigue. Items are rated on a 5-point scale indicating how true each statement was for the respondent in the previous week. One can merge the FSI intensity, FSI frequency, and MSFI scores to provide a comprehensive fatigue composite, provided the resulting $\alpha > .80$, indicating good internal consistency.

Benefit Finding

We have also included a measure to assess benefit finding (i.e., whether participants think they have benefited from the experience of being diagnosed with and treated for breast cancer). This measure was derived from several sources, including an item set by Behr, Murphy, and Summers (1992) designed to assess perceptions of benefit finding among parents of children with special needs. Several of the items were refocused so that they were applicable to breast cancer, and additional items were created. We condensed the item set by removing items endorsed infrequently and those that seemed redundant, resulting in a 17-item measure referred to as the Benefit Finding Scale (BFS; Antoni, Lehman, Boyers, et al., 2001). Each item begins with the phrase "Having had breast cancer has . . . " and ends with some potential benefit that could be derived from the experience. The items assess benefits in various domains, including acceptance of life's imperfections, becoming more cognizant of the role of other people in one's life, and developing a sense of purpose in life. A factor analysis of responses from the initial assessment suggests the measure is appropriately used as a unitary scale. The average internal reliability (across the four assessments) of the item set in one study was .95.

ABBREVIATED BATTERY

Clinicians who would like to use an abbreviated battery of tests to assess progress during the B-SMART intervention may decide to use the BDI or CES–D to measure depressive symptoms, the POMS as a general distress measure, and the SIP as a preliminary index of quality of life. Those interested in assessing participant changes in perceived benefits could add the BFS to this battery. This battery is brief, is sensitive to changes in the nonclinical range, and can be administered as a questionnaire or as an interview when necessary. Although comparative norms and clinical cutoff scores are available for the BDI, changes in the POMS, the BFS and SIP need to be evaluated on an individual basis.

B-SMART INTERVENTION TARGETS: MEDIATORS OF THERAPEUTIC CHANGE

Our theoretical model specifies a set of variables that are conceptually related to the major goals of the B-SMART intervention and may mediate the changes in outcome measures that are observed during the program. In keeping with the goals and strategies of the program, these intervention targets are represented by measures of cognitive appraisals, coping strategies and coping self-efficacy, social support, and emotional processing. From a clinical standpoint, this information may also provide information about differences in the ways that this intervention benefits different participants.

Cognitive Appraisals

We have used the Dysfunctional Attitude Scale (DAS; Weissman & Beck, 1978) to measure changes in maladaptive or dysfunctional cognitive appraisals and attitudes among B-SMART participants. The DAS is a 100-item self-report inventory that uses a 7-point Likert scale. Higher scores indicate a greater number of cognitive distortions. We have found that higher DAS scores are associated with a greater use of maladaptive HIV-specific coping strategies such as denial and behavioral disengagement and less use of more adaptive strategies such as active coping and seeking social support among people in a CBSM intervention (Penedo et al., 2001). Greater decreases in DAS scores were also related to greater reductions in depressive symptoms and general distress levels among CBSM participants (Cruess, Antoni, Hayes, et al., 2002). Clinicians may find the DAS useful for gauging treatment progress and may also find it helpful to observe changes in specific cognitive distortions that are more salient for particular individuals.

Coping Strategies

We have used the situational version of the COPE (Carver et al., 1989) to measure changes in specific coping strategies (e.g., strategies used to deal with breast cancer and its treatment) during the intervention. Though originally developed as a 57-item inventory, a newer 24-item version of the COPE is now available. Clinicians can administer the COPE before and after the B-SMART program and ask patients to make their responses global (i.e., about life in general) or specific (i.e., about challenges specific to breast cancer). Based on our previous work, the COPE scales most applicable to changes that occur during the B-SMART program include those that describe active/involvement strategies (e.g., active coping, planning, positive reframing, acceptance, seeking emotional support, seeking instrumental support) and those that describe denial/disengagement strategies (e.g., denial, mental disengagement, behavioral disengagement). Active/involvement strategies are those used to actively involve oneself and one's resources in managing stressors. Some of these strategies are more behavioral (e.g., active coping, planning), others are more cognitive (e.g., positive reframing, acceptance), and still others are more interpersonal (e.g., seeking social support). Less adaptive forms of coping are indexed with denial/disengagement strategies, strategies that are designed to distance the person from or deny the existence of stressors. These strategies include mental and behavioral forms of disengagement from stress and outright denial of the source of stress. One major goal of the program is to help participants increase their use of active/involvement strategies and decrease the use of less adaptive denial/disengagement strategies, with the hopes that this will decrease distress levels and depressive symptoms.

Coping Self-Efficacy

An important set of skills that we hope B-SMART participants will develop is stress management skills. We have previously measured these skills with the 6-item Coping Self-Efficacy (CSE) scale, a measure developed during our previous work with gay men who were infected with HIV (Ironson et al., 1994). We have tailored this measure to evaluate B-SMART participants' perceived efficacy in managing future cancer-specific symptoms and stressors by using various CBSM strategies such as relaxation and cognitive restructuring. We recently created a more extensive instrument, the Measure of Current Status (MOCS; Carver & Antoni, 1999), which includes brief sets of items used to measure participants' current self-perceived status with respect to the ability to relax at will, the ability to recognize stress-inducing situations, the ability to stop and restructure maladaptive thoughts, the ability to be assertive about needs, the ability to express anger effectively and appropriately, the ability to call on social support when needed, and the ability to choose appropriate coping responses when needed, as well as related changes in areas such as feelings of normalcy versus alienation related to being treated for cancer, a sense of cohesiveness with other patients with cancer, perceptions of attention coming from people around them (including but not limited to the group), and a sense of being better off than other patients with cancer. Many of these are targets of intervention modules; others are potential nonspecific effects, or by-products, of the intervention. All these elements can be influenced by experiences outside the intervention as well. The items are appropriate for participants in B-SMART and for isolation of *critical elements predicting well-being,* regardless of whether the elements are acquired during the intervention.

Social Support

Changes in qualitative aspects of social support during the B-SMART program can be measured with the Social Provisions Scale (SPS; Cutrona & Russell, 1987), a 24-item self-report questionnaire. This instrument measures perceived social support using several domains, including social integration, reassurance of worth, attachment, opportunities for nurturance, reliable alliance, and guidance—all of which are hypothesized to be associated with the protective effects of social relationships (Sarason, 1979). We have found that CBSM participants show significant changes in many of these dimensions, especially attachment, guidance, and reliable alliance (Lutgendorf et al., 1998). At the beginning and end of the B-SMART program, we also administer other assessments to measure changes in participants' sources of social support (e.g., friends, family, professionals) and their degree of satisfaction with the support. These sources can vary significantly across and within populations. For example, in a study of gay men with HIV, we found that the men relied on their friends as a source of support nearly twice as often as they relied on family members and nearly ten times more often than they relied on professional support providers (Zuckerman, 1995). Nevertheless, these sources of support are likely to vary widely among different individuals, and even slight changes in scores during the course of the intervention can be clinically meaningful. For instance, increases in previously unused sources of support may signal important treatment gains.

Emotional Processing

In our work, we have also included a measure of emotional processing (Stanton et al., 2000). This scale contains two sets of items, one on examination of emotions (e.g., *I've been taking time to figure out what I'm really feeling, I've been exploring my emotions*), another on expression of emotions (e.g., *I've been expressing the feelings I am having, I've been taking time to express my emotions*). Responses are made on a scale with the following labels: *I haven't been doing this at all* (a), *I've been doing this a little bit* (b), *I've been doing this a medium amount* (c), and *I've been doing this a lot* (d). Clinicians can use these scales to explore one aspect of the processes we expect to be induced by the intervention—those related to emotional awareness and expression. Thus, the scales can be used to check on an aspect of the "process" impact of the intervention. We have found significant increases in this measure during the 10-week B-SMART program (Antoni et al., 2001).

ABBREVIATED BATTERY

Clinicians using the B-SMART intervention may decide to use an abbreviated battery of intervention target assessments that includes the COPE, the CSE, and the SPS. Although these measures do not document changes in the ultimate outcomes for the intervention (i.e., distress reduction), they do provide insight into the process variables that may underlie the ultimate clinical gains and can be used to detect areas in which participants may need additional help.

PHYSICAL HEALTH-RELATED MEASURES

The health-related assessments that we have used to evaluate the effects of the B-SMART program include immunological assays, hormonal measures, and measures based on physical health symptoms. Although these measurements are certainly not necessary for clinicians using this program, this information may help clinicians explain to medical centers or multidisciplinary services that these measures should be timed so that they can assess pretreatment and posttreatment changes.

The number of these sorts of measures that are used may have to be limited according to cost considerations and logistics. In some cases, the assessments can be "piggybacked" onto participants' preexisting and scheduled physical examinations and blood tests to assess pretreatment and posttreatment changes. Other more time-sensitive measures may need to be more carefully controlled and are best assessed in the same laboratory with the same internal standards and reagents. For instance, indexes such as natural killer cell cytotoxicity (NKCC) and 24-hour urinary catecholamine measures, which are acutely sensitive to changes in stress (and posture) levels and varying in a diurnal fashion, must be measured shortly before the commencement and completion of the program, at the same time of day, and with commensurate measurements of acute mood state at the time of venipuncture. Other measures such as lymphocyte cell counts and other laboratory progression markers (e.g., CA-15, vascular endothelial growth factor) change more slowly and could be collected at regular clinic visits before and after the B-SMART intervention, provided that the tests are conducted in the same laboratory.

Specific Immune System Measures

Numerous immunological measures (and multiple assay systems for each of these) are currently available for describing changes in quantitative (e.g., lymphocyte cell counts) and qualitative (e.g., proliferation, cytotoxicity, antibody production, cytokine production) aspects of the immune system. Recent positive trends in the measurement technologies available for psychoneuroimmunology research include the use of antigen-specific functional assays (e.g., antigen-specific cytotoxicity tests that use breast cancer–associated cell lines) and stimulated, or "enhanced," function tests (e.g., mitogen-induced cytokine production by lymphocytes, cytokine-enhanced NKCC using recombinant interleukin-2 [IL-2] or interferon-gamma [IFN-γ]). Although many of these tests have been widely used in animal studies, they have not been widely used in studies of breast cancer in humans (e.g., Andersen et al., 1998). It is unlikely that research will identify a single immune measure that is an indicator of long-term health in patients with breast cancer, thus researchers track patterns of changes in several indicators.

Because many of these immune measures are affected by disease stage and treatment, one strategy for tracking immune system changes during psychosocial intervention is to restrict studies to patients with a specific stage (or range of stages) of the disease (e.g., breast cancer stages I, II, and III) and to have blood samples taken before and after the period of adjuvant chemotherapy, radiation, or immunotherapy. For these reasons, we have been monitoring a specific set of immune measures before and at a follow-up point after the B-SMART intervention period among women diagnosed with stages I, II, or II breast cancer. We begin monitoring 4 to 8 weeks after surgery but before the onset of chemotherapy or radiation therapy. We draw the postintervention blood samples 3 months after the conclusion of the intervention, when adjuvant therapy has (in most cases) been completed. We continue to monitor the women at regular time intervals to assess the short-term (e.g., 3 months) and longer term (e.g., 9 months) effects of the intervention on immune variables that may predict retarded disease progression and relapse several years later.

For our assessment battery, we chose specific immunological measures that have previously been shown to relate to our psychosocial outcome variables. Impairments in NKCC and lymphocyte proliferative responses to mitogens are related to depressive symptoms (Irwin, Patterson, et al., 1990) and uncontrollable life events such as bereavement (Irwin, Caldwell, et al., 1990). A comprehensive assessment of immune system status in patients with breast cancer going through the B-SMART program might include (a) lymphocyte cell counts and subpopulations of cells with specific functions, (b) immune system functions such as NKCC and lymphocyte proliferative responses, (c) immune system chemical mediators such as the T-helper-type-1 (Th1) cytokines IL-2 and IFN-γ and T-helper-type-2 (Th2) cytokines IL-4 and IL-10. This battery of tests may be very expensive to administer and should be created in close collaboration with an immunologist with relevant cancer experience.

Neuroendocrine Measures

To better understand the potential mediators of psychoimmune interactions, it is useful to assess neurohormones associated with sympathetic nervous system (SNS) activation (catecholamines such as epinephrine and norepinephrine), the hypothalamic–pituitary–adrenocortical (HPAC) system (cortisol, adrenocorticotrophic hormone; ACTH), and endorphins, prolactin, and numerous additional substances (Meier, Watkins, & Fleishner, 1994). Assays are available for monitoring these substances in the blood, urine, and in some cases, saliva. Decisions regarding the sampling compartment of choice depend on the time frame that is being evaluated. Neurohormones are important regulators of the magnitude and timing of the immune system's response to stressful stimuli; researchers have more to learn about the relevance and temporality of immunological and neurohormone responses to standardized challenges as they relate to emotional responses to stressful stimuli or related events. For instance, it would be interesting to examine whether individual differences in emotional resolution of stressful stimuli or traumatic events in the environment are reflected in a faster immunological and neurohormonal "recovery" from standardized laboratory challenges such as solving mental arithmetic problems or public speaking (Starr et al., 1996). Once these parallels are established, it may be possible to develop designs that use laboratory challenges for assessing physiological response efficiency before and after psychological or pharmacological intervention in patients with breast cancer (van der Pompe et al., 2001). Another advantage of using hormonal assessments to evaluate changes in psychosocial intervention programs is that these types of measurements may provide a more valid picture of psychological distress levels than self-reports, which may be affected by social desirability and selective recall biases.

We have used a relatively basic neuroendocrine battery in the studies evaluating the effects of CBSM intervention. These tests focus specifically on 24-hour urinary catecholamine levels (epinephrine and norepinephrine) and cortisol levels, as well as plasma measured in the week before and just after the CBSM intervention program (Antoni, Cruess, Cruess, et al., 2000; Antoni, Cruess, Wagner, et al., 2000; Cruess, Antoni, Schneiderman, et al., 2000). For the urinary assessments, participants are required to collect and store their urine for a full 24 hours before their assessment visit and to then bring the urine collection container to our assessment core laboratory, from which it is sent to a biochemistry lab for analysis. For some participants who are employed in full-time jobs, it may not be ideal to collect urine during the entire 24-hour cycle. It is possible to have these participants limit their urine collection to hours when they are not working (e.g., 6:00 p.m. to 9:00 a.m.). These 15-hour intervals must be maintained at each measurement point if hormonal values are to be compared over time.

Special care must be taken to provide participants with detailed written instructions concerning collection and sample storage procedures and dietary and substance restrictions they must be adhere to during the collection period. Some of these restrictions may make it unfeasible for certain participants to provide this type of information. For these participants, it might be better to collect blood or salivary samples at the time of the assessment visit, and the hormones can be assayed from these samples. We have used afternoon blood samples collected before and immediately after the 10-week B-SMART program to document significant reductions in cortisol level during the intervention period (D. Cruess, Antoni, McGregor, et al., 2000). We have also used saliva samples collected within our weekly CBSM sessions in other populations to assess relaxation-induced changes in cortisol levels and map these out during the 10 weeks of the intervention (D. Cruess, Antoni, Kumar, & Schneiderman, 2000). Salivary cortisol assays appear to be very sensitive to relaxation-induced changes and are also associated with changes in mood states such as anxiety.

However, although salivary and plasma- or serum-derived neuroendocrine measures are useful for monitoring short-term task-induced changes, urinary cortisol and catecholamine (e.g., whole-body 24-hour catecholamine output) levels provide better integrated measures of levels during periods of days. A novel measurement strategy now involves collecting multiple saliva samples during the day to assess total cortisol output as well as individual differences in diurnal fluctuations before and after the intervention. Interestingly, some evidence suggests that altered cortisol output levels during the day may predict differences in survival time among patients with breast cancer (Spiegel, Sephton, Terr, & Stites, 1998). Clinicians considering a neuroendocrine measure to be used for tracking progress in the B-SMART program should consult with a biochemist or endocrinologist as they choose the best overall measure. Generally, cortisol is one of the easiest and least expensive of the stress hormones to assay, less sensitive to momentary fluctuations than others hormones such as catecholamines, and the most resilient to temperature changes that may occur before and during cold storage.

Other Intercurrent Medical and Health Behavior Measurements

It may be interesting to measure other background variables that could affect the course of treatment, including intercurrent life changes related to medical service use and medication changes; changes in substance use and sexual behaviors; exercise, sleep, and diet changes; and major life events and hassles. Any of these factors could improve or hinder treatments, possibly reducing, masking, or amplifying changes in outcomes and targets during the intervention period. Clinicians may find that the recurrence of some negative health behavior (e.g., substance use) may be hindering patients' progress in their stress management activities. In a situation such as this, the treatment plan can be adjusted so that it focuses more on the behavior problem before the patient continues to learn more stress management techniques. Alternatively, clinicians may observe that decreases in distress and depression levels resulting from participation in the B-SMART program may be accompanied by reductions in negative health behaviors (e.g., decreased substance use, increased medical regimen adherence). Documenting such changes may be helpful for clinicians who need to justify the use of the program in certain medical settings where these sorts of behaviors can compromise medical management and increase costs.

Assessment of Patient Satisfaction

At the end of each weekly B-SMART session, we give participants the opportunity to complete an evaluation sheet that focuses specifically on the materials covered in that particular session. This evaluation sheet provides us with information regarding the degree to which participants experience reductions in stress and tension during the session and gives them the opportunity to indicate which procedures they did or did not find useful that day. Occasionally, group members will indicate that they are experiencing some difficulty with one or two procedures introduced during a particular group session. Although participants may feel uncomfortable announcing such difficulties to other group members, they often will indicate such problems on the evaluation sheet. Therefore, reviewing evaluation sheets may help group leaders determine which problems are being experienced by various participants and may result in a productive group discussion (or individual discussion if necessary) the following week. Such information allows clinicians to structure the group in a way that allows them to address important issues and maximize the benefits of the program for participants.

Recommendations for Extension of B-SMART Validation Studies to Other Populations

A prior section of this volume describes in detail the results of studies that evaluated the effects of psychosocial factors on women's adjustment to breast cancer diagnosis and treatment and studies demonstrating the efficacy of the B-SMART program with these women. In brief, these findings suggest that this intervention reduces distress and depression and normalizes some aspects of endocrine and immune system functioning in women during the stressful period after surgery. We are now examining whether changes in these psychosocial factors predict disease progression and quality of life for longer periods. We designed the B-SMART program so that it would be useful for a wide variety of individuals affected by breast cancer. However, the studies completed to date have been limited to people who are in the early to middle stages of the disease in the weeks after surgery (lumpectomy or mastectomy). We are currently testing whether this intervention is effective in improving adjustment in women in a similar disease stage who are just completing adjuvant therapy and have somewhat different psychological challenges. Because patients with advanced disease (i.e., metastatic breast cancer) very likely have additional issues to address, we are going to conduct pilot studies to identify these issues and how well the B-SMART components can address them. We are also studying how the B-SMART intervention affects social support and conflict resolution interactions between patients with breast cancer and their primary partners. We are videotaping the couples' interactions before and after the completion of the 10-week program.

Until just a few years ago, the majority of the studies examining psychosocial factors in patients with breast cancer focused on White middle-class women. One ongoing issue involves the generalizability of such intervention effects to ethnic minorities such as Hispanic, Asian, African American, Native American, and other ethnic minority women with breast cancer. Researchers are beginning to realize that these groups experience many of the same psychosocial sequelae of breast cancer diagnosis and treatment as do White women, but the issues are compounded by extreme financial burdens, social isolation, and a lack of access to support services and support groups, especially among those of lower socioeconomic status. Some of these women also have additional issues such as drug and alcohol dependency, numerous medical problems that are not related to cancer, and a general feeling of powerlessness. Because of the alarming increase in the incidence of breast cancer in ethnic minority women who live in the inner city, we have made numerous attempts to test the effects of B-SMART on African American women and Spanish-speaking Latina women with breast cancer. A Spanish translation of the *Participant's Workbook* for B-SMART has just been completed and was designed to be sensitive to cultural issues involving cancer and cancer treatment. We are in the process of conducting efficacy trials of this version of the intervention. Although we have modified some aspects of the procedures for implementing the B-SMART sessions with these populations, all of the techniques and therapy format parameters have been matched with those used in our prior and ongoing studies, which will allow us to compare the relative effectiveness of the program for different populations of people who have breast cancer. Although we have not conducted any analyses of the relative effectiveness of the B-SMART program among different ethnic groups it is plausible that the program may have different effects among these groups because of differences in (a) the ways they perceive illness in general, (b) the ways they have developed to deal with or deny the cancer diagnosis, (c) the ways they experience the treatment process, and (d) how comfortable and willing they are to share information in a group setting with women they perceive to be more or less like themselves. As we attempt to improve the effectiveness of the B-SMART program, we will need to take these factors into consideration during studies of African American, Asian American, and Native American women.

Recommendations for Systematic Evaluations Across Sites

The APA Task Force on Psychological Intervention Guidelines noted the importance of coordinating the evaluation programs of different clini-

T A B L E   5 . 2

Suggested Measures for Monitoring Progress in the B-SMART Program in Different Treatment and Research Settings

Domain	Minimal clinical assessment	Extended clinical assessment	System/program evaluation	Validation/replication research
Screening	Intake interview	Intake interview	SCID MMSE MBMD	SCID SCID–II SIGH–AD MMSE MBMD
Adherence	Group attendance	Group attendance	Group attendance	Group attendance
Skill acquisition	PMR: home practice, *Participant's Workbook* assignments	PMR: home practice, within-session POMS	PMR: home practice, PMR: behavioral rating, *Participant's Workbook* assignments	Workbook homework, within-session POMS, *Participant's Workbook* assignments
Treatment outcome	CES–D	CES–D	CES–D SF–36 POMS BFS	CES–D POMS SF–36 SIP IES BFS
Intervention targets	—	COPE CSE/MOCS SPS	COPE CSE/MOCS SPS EPS	COPE CSE/MOCS DAS SPS SSSS EPS

Note. SCID = Structured Clinical Interview for *DSM–IV*; SCID–II = Structured Clinical Interview for *DSM–IV* Axis II personality disorders; SIGH–AD = Structured Interview Guide for Hamilton Anxiety and Depression; MMSE = Mini Mental Status Exam; PMR = progressive muscle relaxation; POMS = Profile of Mood States; SF–36 = Health Status Questionnaire—Short Form; SIP = Sickness Impact Profile; IES = Impact of Event Scale; DAS = Dysfunctional Attitudes Scale; SPS = Social Provisions Scale; SSSS = Source of Social Support Scale; CSE = Coping Self-Efficacy Scale; MOCS = Measure of Current Status; EPS = Emotional Processing Scale; MBMD = Millon Behavioral Medicine Diagnostic.

cians who are using standardized intervention programs (APA, 1995). As discussed in the opening paragraph of this chapter, collecting systematic evaluations of intervention efficacy would allow clinicians to create a cumulative database of assessments that could ultimately facilitate a systematic review of experimental replications through sophisticated techniques such as meta-analysis. A large sample would allow clinicians to address the issue of patient/treatment matching—specifically, individual-differences variables (e.g., personality, demographic, medical) that predict optimal responses to a given intervention such as the B-SMART program. Therefore, it is essential that the assessment battery chosen by clinicians for evaluating intervention efficacy include both measures that are sensitive to change over time (i.e., pretreatment, posttreatment, follow-up) and those that can characterize factors that address patient/treatment matching and generalizability issues. In Table 5.2, we summarize several of the assessment techniques used in the development and initial evaluations of the B-SMART program and include suggestions for different abbreviated batteries (according to the specific goals) in the hopes that users of this intervention program will contribute to the process of systematic evaluation. The different assessment settings addressed by Table 5.2 range from a minimal clinical assessment that could be used by private practitioners to a comprehensive assessment battery that could be used in a funded research project designed to validate or replicate the B-SMART program in different clinical populations.

References

Adler, N., Horowitz, M., Garcia, A., & Moyer, A. (1998). Additional validation of a scale to assess positive states of mind. *Psychosomatic Medicine, 60,* 26–32.

Affleck, G., & Tennen, H. (1996). Construing benefits from adversity: Adaptational significance and disposition underpinnings. *Journal of Personality, 64,* 899–922.

Agarwal, S. K., & Marshall, G. D., Jr. (1998). Glucocorticoid-induced type 1/type 2 cytokine alterations in humans: A model for stress-related immune dysfunction. *Journal of Interferon Cytokine Research, 18,* 1059–1068.

Aizawa, K., Ueki, K., Suzuki, S., Yabusaki, H., Kanda, T., Nishimaki, T., et al. (1999). Apoptosis and *bcl-2* expression in gastric carcinomas: Correlation with clinicopathological variables, *p53* expression, cell proliferation and prognosis. *International Journal of Oncology, 14,* 85–91.

Aldwin, C. M., Sutton, K. J., & Lachman, M. (1996). The development of coping resources in adulthood. *Journal of Personality, 64,* 837–871.

Aleo, S., & Nicassio, P. (1978). *Auto-regulation of duodenal ulcer disease: A preliminary report of four cases.* Proceedings of the Ninth Annual Meeting of the Bio-feedback Society of America, Denver, CO.

Alferi, S., Antoni, M. H., Ironson, G., Kilbourn, K., & Carver, C. S. (2001). Factors predicting the use of complementary therapies in a multi-ethnic sample of early-stage breast cancer patients. *Journal of the American Medical Women's Association, 56,* 120–126.

Alferi, S., Carver, C. S., Antoni, M. H., Weiss, S., & Duran, R. (2001). An exploratory study of social support, distress, and disruption among low-income Hispanic women under treatment for early-stage breast cancer. *Health Psychology, 20,* 41–46.

Alferi, S., Culver, J., Carver, C. S., Arena, P., & Antoni, M. H. (1999). Religiosity, religious coping, and distress: A prospective study of Catholic and evangelical Hispanic women in treatment for early stage breast cancer. *Journal of Health Psychology, 4,* 343–356.

Altare, F., Lammas, D., Emile, J. F., Lamhamedi, S., Le Deist, F., Drysdale, P., et al. (1998). Impairment of mycobacterial immunity in human interleukin-12 receptor deficiency. *Science, 280,* 1432–1435.

American Psychological Association. (1995). *Template for developing guidelines: Inter-*

ventions for mental disorders and psychosocial aspects of physical disorders. Washington, DC: Author.

Amsterdam, J. D., Maislin, G., Gold, P., & Winkour, A. (1989). The assessment of abnormalities in hormonal responsiveness at multiple levels of the hypothalamic–pituitary–adrenocortical axis in depressive illness. *Psychoneuroendocrinology, 14*(1–2), 43–62.

Andersen, B. (1992). Psychological interventions for cancer patients to enhance the quality of life. *Journal of Consulting and Clinical Psychology, 60*, 552–568.

Andersen, B. (1998, August). *Stress, immune and endocrine responses following a psychological intervention for women with regional breast cancer.* Paper presented at the International Congress of Behavioral Medicine, Copenhagen, Denmark.

Andersen, B., Farrar, W., Golden-Kreutz, D., Kutz, L., MacCallum, R., Courtney, M., et al. (1998). Stress and immune responses after surgical treatment for regional breast cancer. *Journal of the National Cancer Institute, 90*, 30–36.

Andersen, B., Golden-Kreutz, D., & Farrar, W. (1997, November). *Stress reduction and enhanced coping from a psychological/behavioral intervention for women with regional breast cancer: Studies from the stress and immunity breast cancer project.* Paper presented at the Era of Hope meeting of the Department of Defense Breast Cancer Research Program, Washington, DC.

Andersen, B., Kiecolt-Glaser, J., & Glaser, R. (1994). A biobehavioral model of cancer stress and disease course. *American Psychologist, 49*, 389–404.

Andrasik, F., Blanchard, E. B., Neff, D. F., & Rodichok, L. D. (1984). Biofeedback and relaxation training for chronic headache: A controlled comparison of booster treatments and regular contacts for long-term maintenance. *Journal of Consulting and Clinical Psychology, 52*, 609–615.

Antoni, M. H. (1987). Neuroendocrine influences in psychoimmunology and neoplasia: A review. *Psychology and Health, 1*, 3–24.

Antoni, M. H. (1997). Cognitive behavioral stress management for gay men learning of their HIV-1 antibody test results. In J. Spira (Ed.), *Group therapy for patients with chronic medical diseases* (pp. 55–91). New York: Guilford Press.

Antoni, M. H. (1997). Emotional disclosure in the face of stress: Physiological correlates. In. A Vingerhoets, F. van Bussel, & J. Boelhouwer (Eds.), *The (non) expression of emotions in health and disease.* Tilburg, Netherlands: Tilburg University Press.

Antoni, M. H., Baggett, L., Ironson, G., August, S., LaPerriere, A., Klimas, N., et al. (1991). Cognitive–behavioral stress management intervention buffers distress responses and immunologic changes following notification of HIV-1 seropositivity. *Journal of Consulting and Clinical Psychology, 6*, 906–915.

Antoni, M. H., Cruess, D., Wagner, S., Lutgendorf, S., Kumar, M., Ironson, G., et al. (2000). Cognitive–behavioral stress management effects on anxiety, 24-hour urinary catecholamine output, and T-cytotoxic/suppressor cells over time among symptomatic HIV-infected gay men. *Journal of Consulting and Clinical Psychology, 68*, 31–45.

Antoni, M. H., Cruess, S., Cruess, D., Kumar, M., Lutgendorf, S., Ironson, G., et al. (2000). Cognitive–behavioral stress management reduces distress and 24-hour urinary free cortisol among symptomatic HIV-infected gay men. *Annals of Behavioral Medicine, 22*, 1–11.

Antoni, M. H., & Goodkin, K. (1996). Cervical neoplasia, human papillomavirus and psychoneuroimmunology. In H. Friedman & A. Friedman (Eds.), *Psychoneuroimmunology and infectious disease* (pp. 243–262). Boca Raton, FL: CRC Press.

Antoni, M. H., Lehman, J., Kilbourn, K., Boyers, A., Yount, S., Culver, J., et al. (2001). Cognitive–behavioral stress management intervention decreases the prevalence of depression and enhances benefit finding among women under treatment for early-stage breast cancer. *Health Psychology, 20*, 20–32.

Antoni, M. H., Wagner, S., Cruess, D., Kumar, M., Lutgendorf, S., Ironson, G., et al. (2000). Cognitive behavioral stress management reduces distress and 24-hour urinary free cortisol among symptomatic HIV-infected gay men. *Annals of Behavioral Medicine, 22*, 29–37.

Awwad, M., & North, R. J. (1990). Radiosensitive barrier to T-cell-mediated adoptive immunotherapy of established tumors. *Cancer Research, 50,* 2228–2233.

Axelrod, J., & Reisine, T. D. (1984). Stress hormones: Their interaction and regulation. *Science, 224,* 452–459.

Baider, L., Uziely, B., & De-Nour, A. (1994). Progressive muscle relaxation and guided imagery in cancer patients. *General Hospital Psychiatry, 16,* 340–347.

Bandura, A. (1986). *Social foundations of thought and action: A social cognitive theory.* Englewood Cliffs, NJ: Prentice-Hall.

Barraclough, J., Pinder, P., Cruddas, M., Osmond, C., Taylor, I., & Perry, M. (1992). Life events and breast cancer prognosis. *British Medical Journal, 304,* 1078–1081.

Bartlett, E. (1983). Educational self-help approaches in childhood asthma. *Journal of Allergy and Clinical Immunology, 72,* 545–554.

Baum, A., McKinnon, Q., & Silvia, C. (1987). *Chronic stress and the immune system.* Paper presented at the meeting of the Society of Behavioral Medicine, New York, NY.

Baum, A., & Posluszny, D. (1999). Health psychology: Mapping biobehavioral contributions to health and illness. *Annual Review of Psychology, 50,* 137–163.

Baumstark, K., & Beck, N. (1988). *A cognitive–behavioral treatment package for management of postoperative cesarean-section pain.* Paper presented at the ninth annual Scientific Sessions of the Society of Behavioral Medicine, Boston, MA.

Baxevanis, C., Reclos, G., Gritzapis, A., Dedousis, G., Missitzis, I., & Papamichail, M. (1993). Elevated prostaglandin E2 production by monocytes is responsible for the depressed levels of natural killer and lymphokine-activated killer cell function in patients with breast cancer. *Cancer, 72,* 491–501.

Beck, A., & Emery, G. (1979). *Cognitive therapy of anxiety and phobic disorders.* Philadelphia: Center for Cognitive Therapy.

Beck, A., Rush, A., Shaw, B., & Emery, G. (1979). *Cognitive therapy of depression.* New York: Guilford Press.

Beck, A. I., Ward, C. H., Mendelson, M., Mock, J., & Erbaugh, J. (1961). An inventory for measuring depression. *Archives of General Psychiatry, 4,* 561–571.

Behr, S. K., Murphy, D. L., & Summers, J. A. (1992). *User's manual: Kansas Inventory of Parental Perceptions.* Lawrence: University of Kansas, Beach Center on Families and Disabilities.

Berglund, G., Bolund, G., Gustafsson, U., & Sjoden, P. (1994). A randomized study of a rehabilitation program for cancer patients: The "starting again" group. *Psycho-Oncology, 3,* 109–120.

Bergner, M., Bobbitt, R. A., Carter, W. B., & Gilson, B. S. (1981). The Sickness Impact Profile: Development and final revision of a health status measure. *Medical Care, 19,* 787–806.

Bernstein, B., & Borkovec, T. (1973). *Progressive muscle relaxation training: A manual for the helping professions.* Champaign, IL: Research Press.

Berrino, F., Muti, P., Micheli, A., Bolelli, G., Krogh, V., Sciajno, R., et al. (1996). Serum sex hormone levels after menopause and subsequent breast cancer. *Journal of the National Cancer Institute, 88,* 291–296.

Besedovsky, H., del Rey, A., Sorkin, E., DaPrada, M., Burri, R., & Honegger, C. (1983). The immune response evokes changes in brain noradrenergic neurons. *Science, 221,* 564–565.

Blackburn, I., & Bishop, S. (1983). Changes in cognition with pharmacotherapy and cognitive therapy. *British Journal of Psychiatry, 143,* 609–617.

Blackburn, I., Jones, S., & Lewin, R. (1986). Cognitive style in depression. *Clinical Psychology, 25,* 241–251.

Blalock, J. E., Bost, K. L., & Smith, E. M. (1985). Neuroendocrine peptide hormones and their receptors in the immune system. Production, processing, and action. *Journal of Neuroimmunology, 10,* 31–40.

Bloom, J. R. (1982). Social support, accommodation to stress, and adjustment to breast cancer. *Social Science and Medicine, 16,* 1329–1338.

Bloom, J. R. (1986). Social support and adjustment to breast cancer. In B. L. Andersen (Ed.), *Women with cancer: Psychological perspectives.* New York: Springer-Verlag.

Bloom, J. R. (1987). Psychological response to mastectomy: A prospective comparison study. *Cancer, 59,* 189–196.

Bolger, N., Foster, M., Vinokur, A., & Ng, R. (1996). Close relationships and adjustment to a life crisis: The case of breast cancer. *Journal of Personality and Social Psychology, 70,* 283–294.

Borkovec, T. D., & Sides, J. K. (1979). Critical procedural variables related to the physiological effects of progressive relaxation: A review. *Behavior, Research, and Therapy, 17,* 119–125.

Bovbjerg, D. (1991). Psychoneuroimmunology: Implications for oncology? *Cancer, 67,* 828–832.

Bovbjerg, D., & Valdimarsdottir, H. (1993). Familial cancer, emotional distress, and low natural cytotoxic activity in healthy women. *Annals of Oncology, 4,* 745–752.

Bovbjerg, D., & Valdimarsdottir, H. (1996). Stress, immune modulation, and infectious disease during chemotherapy for breast cancer. *Annals of Behavioral Medicine, 18,* S63.

Bovbjerg, D., & Valdimarsdottir, H. (1998). Psychoneuroimmunology: Implications for psycho-oncology. In J. Holland (Ed.), *Textbook of psycho-oncology* (pp. 125–134). New York: Oxford University Press.

Brandenburg, Y., Bergenmar, M., & Bjolund, C. (1994). Information to patients with malignant melanoma: A randomized group study. *Patient Educational Counseling, 23,* 97–105.

Brandt, K. (1973). The effects of relaxation training with analog HR feedback on basal levels of arousal and response to aversive tones in groups selected according to Fear Survey scores. *Psychophysiology, 11,* 242.

Breitbart, W., & Mermelstein, H. (1992). An alternative psychostimulant for management of depressive disorders in cancer patients. *Psychosomatics, 33,* 352–356.

Breitbart, W., & Payne, D. (1998). Pain. In J. Holland (Ed.), *Textbook of psycho-oncology* (pp. 450–467). New York: Oxford University Press.

Bridge, L. R., Benson, P., Pietroni, P. C., & Priest, R. G. (1998). Relaxation and imagery in the treatment of breast cancer. *British Medical Journal, 297,* 1169–1172.

Brittenden, J., Heys, S., Ross, J., & Eremin, O. (1996). Natural killer cells and cancer. *Cancer, 77,* 1226–1243.

Brooks, G. R., & Richardson, F. C. (1980). Emotional skills training: A treatment program for duodenal ulcer. *Behavior Therapy, 11,* 198–207.

Brown, J. M. (1984). Imagery coping strategies in the treatment of migraine. *Pain, 18,* 157–167.

Brownell, K., Marlatt, A., Lichenstein, E., & Wilson, G. (1986). Understanding and preventing relapse. *American Psychologist, 41,* 421–438.

Bruckheimer, E. M., Gjertsen, B. T., & McDonnell, T. J. (1999). Implications of cell death regulation in the pathogenesis and treatment of prostate cancer. *Seminars in Oncology, 26,* 382–398.

Bruera, E., Brenneis, C., Paterson, A., & MacDonald, R. (1989). Use of methylphenidate as an adjuvant to narcotic analgesics in patients with advanced cancer. *Journal of Pain Symptom Management, 4,* 3–6.

Buchanan, T. W., al'Absi, M., & Lovallo, W. R. (1999). Cortisol fluctuates with increases and decreases in negative affect. *Psychoneuroendocrinology, 24,* 227–241.

Burns, D. (1981). *Feeling good: The new mood therapy.* New York: New American Library.

Burstein, H. J., Gelber, S., Guadagnoli, E., & Weeks, J. C. (1999). Use of alternative medicine by women with early-stage breast cancer. *New England Journal Medicine, 340,* 1733–1739.

Byrnes, D., Antoni, M., Goodkin, K., Efantis-Potter, J., Simon, T., Munajj, J., et al. (1998). Stressful events, pessimism, natural killer cell cytotoxicity, and cytotoxic/suppressor T-cells in HIV+ Black women at risk for cervical cancer. *Psychosomatic Medicine, 60,* 714–722.

Carroll, B., Curtis, G., & Mendels, J. (1976). Neuroendocrine regulation in depression: I. Limbic system–adrenocortical dysfunction. *Archives of General Psychiatry, 33,* 1034–1044.

Carroll, B., Feinberg, M., Greden, J., Tarika, J., Albala, A., Hasket, R., et al. (1981). A specific laboratory test for the diagnosis of melancholia. *Archives of General Psychiatry, 38,* 15–22.

Carver, C. S., & Antoni, M. H. (1999). The Measure of Current Status (MOCS). Unpublished manuscript, University of Miami, FL.

Carver, C. S., Harris, S., Lehman, J., Durel, J., Antoni, M. H., Spencer, S., et al.

(2000). How important is the perception of personal control? Studies of early stage breast cancer patients. *Personality and Social Psychology Bulletin, 26,* 139–149.

Carver, C. S., Meyer, B., & Antoni, M. H. (2000). Responsiveness to threats and incentives, expectations of cancer recurrence, and the experiences of emotional distress and disengagement: Moderator effects in a sample of early-stage breast cancer patients. *Journal of Consulting and Clinical Psychology, 68,* 965–975.

Carver, C. S., Pozo, C., Harris, S., Noriega, V., Scheier, M., Robinson, D., et al. (1993). How coping mediates the effect of optimism on distress: A study of women with early stage breast cancer. *Journal of Personality and Social Psychology, 65,* 375–390.

Carver, C. S., Pozo-Kaderman, C., Harris, S. D., Noriega, V., Scheier, M. F., Robinson, D. S., et al. (1994). Optimism vs. pessimism predicts the quality of women's adjustment to early stage breast cancer. *Cancer, 73,* 1213–1220.

Carver, C. S., Pozo-Kaderman, C., Price, A. A., Noriega, V., Harris, S. D., Derhagopian, R. P., et al. (1998). Concern about aspects of body image and adjustment to early stage breast cancer. *Psychosomatic Medicine, 60,* 168–174.

Carver, C. S., & Scheier, M. F. (1990). Origins and functions of positive and negative affect: A control-process view. *Psychological Review, 97,* 19–35.

Carver, C. S., & Scheier, M. F. (1998). *On the self-regulation of behavior.* New York: Cambridge University Press.

Carver, C. S., Scheier, M. F., & Weintraub, J. K. (1989). Assessing coping strategies: A theoretically based approach. *Journal of Personality and Social Psychology, 56,* 267–283.

Cauley, J., Lucas, F., Kuller, L., Stone, K., Browner, W., & Cummings, S. (1999). Elevated serum estradiol and testosterone concentrations are associated with a high risk for breast cancer. Study of Osteoporotic Fractures Research Group. *Annals of Internal Medicine, 130*(4, Pt. 1), 270–277.

Cella, D., Tulsky, D., Gray, G., Sarafin, B., Lin, E., Bonomi, A., et al. (1993). The functional assessment of cancer therapy scale: Development and validation of the general measure. *Journal of Clinical Oncology, 11,* 570–579.

Cerottini, J.-C., Lienard, D., & Romero, P. (1996). Recognition of tumor-associated antigens by T-lymphocytes: Perspectives for peptide-based vaccines. *Annals of Oncology, 7,* 339–342.

Christie, J., Whalley, L., Brown, N., & Dick, H. (1982). Effects of ECT on the neuroendocrine response to apomorphine in severely depressed patients. *British Journal of Psychiatry, 140,* 268–273.

Christie, J., Whalley, L., Dick, H., Blackwood, D., Blackburn, I., & Fink, G. (1986). Raised plasma cortisol concentrations a feature of drug-free psychotics and not specific for depression. *British Journal of Psychiatry, 148,* 58–65.

Clark, G., & McGuire, W. (1992). Defining the high-risk breast cancer patient. In I. Henderson (Ed.), *Adjuvant therapy of breast cancer* (pp. 161–187). Norwell, MA: Kluwer Academic.

Classen, C., Sandra, E., Sephton, E., Diamond, S., & Spiegel, D. (1998). Studies of life-extending psychosocial interventions. In J. Holland (Ed.), *Textbook of psycho-oncology* (pp. 730–742). New York: Oxford University Press.

Clerici, M., Merola, M., Ferrario, E., Trabattoni, D., Villa, M. L., Stefanon, B., et al. (1997). Cytokine production patterns in cervical intraepithelial neoplasia: Association with human papillomavirus infection. *Journal of the National Cancer Institute, 89,* 245–250.

Clerici, M., Shearer, G., & Clerici, E. (1998). Cytokine dysregulation in invasive cervical carcinoma and other human neoplasias: Time to consider the TH1/TH2 paradigm. *Journal of the National Cancer Institute, 90,* 261–263.

Cobb, S. (1974). Physiological changes in men whose jobs are abolished. *Journal of Psychosomatic Research, 18,* 245–258.

Cohen, S., & Rabin, B. (1998). Psychologic stress, immunity, and cancer. *Journal of the National Cancer Institute, 90,* 3–4.

Cohen, S., & Syme, S. (1985). *Social support and health.* New York: Academic Press.

Cohen, S., Tyrrell, D., & Smith, A. (1991). Psychological stress in humans and susceptibility to the common cold. *New*

England Journal of Medicine, 325, 606–612.

Coluzzi, P. H., Grant, M., Doroshow, J. H., Rhiner, M., Ferrell, B., & Rivera, L. (1995). Survey of the provision of supportive care services at National Cancer Institute–designated cancer centers. *Journal of Clinical Oncology, 13,* 756–764.

Contreras Ortiz, O., & Stoliar, A. (1988). Immunological changes in human breast cancer. *European Journal of Gynaecological Oncology, 9,* 502–514.

Cordova, M., Studts, J., Hann, D., Jacobsen, P., & Andrykowski, M. (2000). Symptom structure of PTSD following breast cancer. *Journal of Traumatic Stress, 13,* 301–319.

Covi, L., & Lipman, R. (1987). Cognitive behavioral group psychotherapy combined with imipramine in major depression. *Psychopharmacology Bulletin, 23,* 173–176.

Cox, T., & Mackay, C. (1982). Psychosocial factors and psychophysiological mechanisms in the aetiology and development of cancers. *Social Science Medicine, 16,* 381–396.

Crary, B., Borysenko, M., Sutherland, D. C., Kutz, I., Borysenko, J. Z., & Benson, H. (1983). Decrease in mitogen responsiveness of mononuclear cells from peripheral blood after epinephrine administration in humans. *Journal of Immunology, 130,* 694–697.

Crowther, J. H. (1983). Stress management training and relaxation imagery in the treatment of essential hypertension. *Journal of Behavioral Medicine, 6,* 169–187.

Cruess, D., Antoni, M., Cruess, S., Fletcher, M., Ironson, G., Kumar, M., et al. (2000). Cognitive–behavioral stress management increases free testosterone and decreases psychological distress in HIV-seropositive men. *Health Psychology, 19,* 12–20.

Cruess, D., Antoni, M. H., Kumar, M., & Schneiderman, N. (2000). Reductions in salivary cortisol are associated with mood improvement during relaxation training among HIV-1 seropositive men. *Journal of Behavioral Medicine, 23,* 107–122.

Cruess, D., Antoni, M. H., McGregor, B. A., Boyers, A., Kumar, M., Kilbourn, K., et al. (2000). Cognitive–behavioral stress management reduces serum cortisol by enhancing positive contributions among women being treated for early stage breast cancer. *Psychosomatic Medicine, 62,* 304–308.

Cruess, D., Antoni, M. H., McGregor, B., Kilbourn, K., Boyers, A., Alferi, S., et al. (2001). Cognitive behavioral stress management effects on testosterone and positive growth in women with early-stage breast cancer. *International Journal of Behavioral Medicine, 8,* 194–207.

Cruess, D., Antoni, M. H., Schneiderman, N., Ironson, G., Fletcher, M. A., & Kumar, M. (1999). Cognitive–behavioral stress management effects on DHEA-S and serum cortisol in HIV seropositive men. *Psychoneuroendocrinology, 24,* 537–549.

Cruess, D., Antoni, M. H., Schneiderman, N., Ironson, G., McCabe, P., Fernandez, J., et al. (2000). Cognitive behavioral stress management increases free testosterone and decreases psychological distress in HIV seropositive men. *Health Psychology, 19,* 12–20.

Cruess, S., Antoni, M. H., Cruess, D., Fletcher, M. A., Ironson, G., Kumar, M., et al. (2000). Reductions in HSV-2 antibody titers after cognitive–behavioral stress management and relationships with neuroendocrine function, relaxation skills, and social support in HIV+ gay men. *Psychosomatic Medicine, 62,* 828–837.

Cruess, S., Antoni, M. H., Hayes, A., Penedo, F., Ironson, G., et al. (2002). Changes in mood and depressive symptoms and related change processes during cognitive behavioral stress management in HIV-infected men. *Cognitive Therapy and Research, 26,* 373–392.

Cruess, S., Antoni, M. H., Kilbourn, K., Ironson, G., Klimas, N., Fletcher, M., et al. (2000). Optimism, distress and immunologic status in HIV-infected gay men following Hurricane Andrew. *International Journal of Behavioral Medicine, 7,,* 160–182.

Cupps, T. R., & Fauci, A. S. (1982). Neoplasm and systemic vasculitis: A case report. *Arthritis and Rheumatism, 25,* 475–476.

Cutrona, C., & Russell, D. (1987). The provisions of social relationships and adaptation to stress. In W. H. Jones & D. Perlman (Eds.), *Advances in personal relationships* (pp. 37–67). Greenwich, CT: JAI.

Dakof, G., & Taylor, S. (1990). Victims' perceptions of social support: What is helpful from whom? *Journal of Personality and Social Psychology, 58,* 80–89.

Dean, J., Whelan, J., & Meyers, A. (1989). *An incredibly quick way to assess mood states: The incredibly short POMS.* Paper presented at the annual conference of the Association for the Advancement of Applied Sport Psychology. San Antonio, TX.

Derogatis, L. R. (1986). Psychology in cancer medicine: A perspective and overview. *Journal of Consulting and Clinical Psychology, 54,* 632–638.

Derogatis, L., Morrow, G., Fetting, J., Penman, D., Piasetsky, S., Schmale, A., et al. (1983). The prevalence of psychiatric disorders among cancer patients. *Journal of the American Medical Association, 249,* 751–757.

Dishman, R., & Ickes, W. (1981). Self-motivation and adherence to therapeutic exercise. *Journal of Behavioral Medicine, 4,* 421–438.

Dolbeault, S., Szporn, A., & Holland, J. (1999). Psycho-oncology: Where have we been? Where are we going? *European Journal of Cancer, 35,* 1554–1558.

Dow, K., Ferrell, B., Leigh, S., Ly, J., & Gulasekaram, P. (1996). An evaluation of the quality of life among long-term survivors of breast cancer. *Breast Cancer Research and Treatment, 39,* 261–273.

Dranoff, G., Soiffer, R., Lynch, T., Mihm, M., Jung, K., Kolesar, K., et al. (1997). A Phase I study of vaccination with autologous, irradiated melanoma cells engineered to secrete human granulocyte–macrophage colony stimulating factor. *Human Gene Therapy, 8,* 111–123.

Dunkel-Schetter, C. (1984). Social support and cancer: Findings based on patient interviews and their implications. *Journal of Social Issues, 40,* 77–98.

Ebersole, P., & Flores, J. (1989). Positive impact of life crises. *Journal of Social Behavior and Personality, 4,* 463.

Edelman, R. I. (1970). Effects of progressive relaxation on autonomic processes. *Journal of Clinical Psychology, 26,* 421–425.

Edelman, S., Bell, D., & Kidman, A. (1999). A group cognitive behavioural therapy programme with metastatic breast cancer patients. *Psychooncology, 8,* 295–305.

Elenkov, I. J., Papanicolaou, D. A., Wilder, R. L., & Chrousos, G. P. (1996). Modulatory effects of glucocorticoids and catecholamines on human interleukin-12 and interleukin-10 production: Clinical implications. *Proceedings of the Association of American Physicians, 108,* 374–381.

Engstrom, C., Strohl, R., Rose, L., Lewandowski, L., & Stefanek, M. (1999). Sleep alterations in cancer patients. *Cancer Nursing, 22,* 143–148.

Esche, C., Lokshin, A., Shurin, G., Gastman, B., Rabinowich, H., Watkins, S., et al. (1999). Tumor's other immune targets: Dendritic cells. *Journal of Leukocyte Biology, 66,* 336–344.

Esterling, B., Antoni, M. H., Fletcher, M. A., Margulies, S., & Schneiderman, N. (1994). Emotional disclosure through writing or speaking modulates latent Epstein–Barr virus antibody titers. *Journal of Consulting and Clinical Psychology, 62,* 130–140.

Esterling, B., Antoni, M. H., Kumar, M., & Schneiderman, N. (1990). Emotional repression, stress disclosure responses, and Epstein–Barr viral capsid antigen titers. *Psychosomatic Medicine, 52,* 397–410.

Esterling, B., Antoni, M. H., Schneiderman, N., Carver, C., LaPerriere, A., Ironson, G., et al. (1992). Psychosocial modulation of antibody to Epstein–Barr viral capsid antigen and Human Herpes Virus-Type 6 in HIV-1 infected and at-risk gay men. *Psychosomatic Medicine, 54,* 354–371.

Fallowfield, L., & Jenkins, V. (1999). Effective communication skills are the key to good cancer care. *European Journal of Cancer, 35,* 1592–1597.

Fawzy, F., Cousins, N., Fawzy, N., Kemeny, M., Elashoff, R., & Morton, D. (1990). A structured psychiatric intervention for cancer patients. I. Changes over time in methods of coping and affective disturbance. *Archives of General Psychiatry, 47,* 720–728.

Fawzy, I., & Fawzy, N. (1998). Psycho-educational interventions. In J. Holland (Ed.), *Textbook of psycho-oncology* (pp. 676–693). New York: Oxford University Press.

Fawzy, I. F., & Fawzy, N. W., (1996). Psychoeducational interventions. In J. Holland (Ed.), *Textbook of psycho-oncology* (pp. 676–693). New York: Oxford Press.

Fawzy F., Fawzy N., Hyun C., Elashoff, R., Guthrie, D., Fahey, J. L., et al. (1993). Malignant melanoma. Effects of an early structured psychiatric intervention, coping, and affective state on recurrence and survival 6 years later. *Archives of General Psychiatry, 50,* 681–689.

Fawzy, F., Fawzy, N., Hyun, C., & Wheeler, J. (1997). Brief, coping-oriented therapy for patients with malignant melanoma. In J. Spria (Ed.), *Group therapy for medically ill patients* (pp. 133–164). New York: Guilford Press.

Fawzy, F., Kemeny, M., Fawzy, N., Elashoff, R., Morton, D., Cousins, N., et al. (1990). A structured psychiatric intervention for cancer patients: II. Changes over time in immunological measures. *Archives of General Psychiatry, 47,* 729–735.

Feinberg, B. B., Tan, N. S., Gonik, B., Brath, P. C., & Walsh, S. W. (1991). Increased progesterone concentrations are necessary to suppress interleukin-mediated cell cytotoxicity. *American Journal of Obstetrics and Gynecology, 165,* 1872–1876.

Ferrell, B., Dow, K., Leigh, S., Ly, J., & Gulasekaram, P. (1995). Quality of life in long-term cancer survivors. *Oncology Nursing Forum, 22,* 915–922.

Ferrell, B., Grant, M. M., Funk, B., Otis-Green, S., & Garcia, N. (1997). Quality of life in breast cancer survivors as identified by focus groups. *Psycho-Oncology, 6,* 13–23.

Finkel, E. (1999). Does cancer therapy trigger cell suicide? *Science, 286,* 2256–2258.

First, M., Spitzer, R., Gibbons, M., & Williams, J. (1995). *Structured clinical interview for DSM–IV.* New York: Biometrics Research Department.

Fisher, B., Costantino, J. P., Wickerham, D. L., Redmond, C. K., Kavanah, M., Cronin, W. M., et al. (1998). Tamoxifen for prevention of breast cancer: Report of the National Surgical Adjuvant Breast and Bowel Project P-1 Study. *Journal of the National Cancer Institute, 90,* 1371–1388.

Fishman, B., & Loscalzo, M. (1987). Cognitive–behavioral interventions in management of cancer pain: Principles and applications. *Medical Clinics of North America, 71,* 271–287.

Folkman, S. (1984). Personal control and stress and coping processes: A theoretical analysis. *Journal of Personality and Social Psychology, 46,* 839–852.

Folkman, S., Chesney, M., McKusick, L., Ironson, G., Johnson, D., & Coates, T. (1991). Translating coping theory into intervention. In J. Eckenrode (Ed.), *The social context of coping* (pp. 239–259). New York: Plenum.

Folkman, S., & Lazarus, R. (1980). An analysis of coping in a middle-aged community sample. *Journal of Health and Social Behavior, 21,* 219–239.

Folkman, S., Lazarus, R., Gruen, R., & DeLongis, A. (1986). Appraisal, coping, health status, and psychological symptoms. *Journal of Personality and Social Psychology, 50,* 571–579.

Fonteneau, J. F., Le Drean, E., Le Guiner, S., Gervois, N., Diez, E., & Jotereau, F. (1997). Heterogeneity of biologic responses of melanoma-specific CTL. *Journal of Immunology, 15,* 2831–2839.

Forsyth, I. (1991). The mammary gland. *Basic Clinical Endocrinology and Metabolism, 5,* 809–832.

Fox, B. (1998). Psychosocial factors in cancer incidence and prognosis. In J. Holland (Ed.), *Textbook of Psycho-oncology* (pp. 110–124). New York: Oxford University Press.

Fromm, K., Andrykowski, M., & Hunt, J. (1996). Positive and negative psychosocial sequelae of bone marrow transplantation: Implications for quality of life assessment. *Journal of Behavioral Medicine, 19,* 221–240.

Funch, D., & Mettlin, C. (1982). The role of support in relation to recovery from breast surgery. *Social Science and Medicine, 16,* 91–98.

Gabrilovich, D. I., Chen, H. L., Girgis, K. R., Cunningham, H. T., Meny, G. M., Nadaf, S., et al. (1996). Production of vascular endothelial growth factor by human tumors inhibits the functional maturation of dendritic cells. *Nature Medicine, 2,* 1096–1103.

Gall, T., & Evans, D. (1987). The dimensionality of cognitive appraisal and its relationship to physical and psychological well-being. *Journal of Psychology, 12,* 539–546.

Gellert, G., Maxwell, R., & Siegel, B. (1993). Survival of breast cancer patients receiving adjunctive psychosocial support therapy: A 10-year follow-up study. *Journal of Clinical Oncology, 11,* 66–69.

Gerosa, F., Paganin, C., Peritt, D., Paiola, F., Scupoli, M. T., Aste-Amezaga, M., et al. (1996). Interleukin-12 primes human CD4 and CD8 T cell clones for high production of both interferon-gamma and interleukin-10. *Journal of Experimental Medicine, 183,* 2559–2569.

Glaser, R., & Kiecolt-Glaser, J. E. (1994). *Handbook of human stress and immunity.* San Diego, CA: Academic Press.

Glaser, R., Rice, J., Sherida, J., Fertel, R., Stout, J., Speicher, C., et al. (1987). Stress-related immune suppression: Health implications. *Brain, Behavior, and Immunity, 1,* 7–20.

Glaser, R., Rice, J., Speicher, C., Stout, J., & Kiecolt-Glaser, J. (1986). Stress depresses interferon production and natural killer cell activity in humans. *Behavioral Neurosciences, 100,* 675–678.

Glaser, R., Thorn, B., Tarr, K., Kiecolt-Glaser, J., & D'Ambrosio, S. (1985). Effects of stress on methyltransferase synthesis: An important DNA repair enzyme. *Health Psychology, 4,* 403–412.

Gold, P., Loriaux, D., Roy, A., Kling, M., Calabrese, J., Kellner, C., et al. (1986). Response to corticotropin-releasing hormone in the hypercortisolism of depression and Cushing's disease. *New England Journal of Medicine, 314,* 1329–1335.

Goldstein, I. B., Shapiro, D., & Thananopavarn, C. (1984). Home relaxation techniques for essential hypertension. *Psychosomatic Medicine, 46,* 398–414.

Goodkin, K., Blaney, N., Feaster, D., & Fletcher, M. A. (1992). Active coping is associated with natural killer cell cytotoxicity in asymptomatic HIV-1 seropositive homosexual men. *Journal of Psychosomatic Research, 36,* 635–650.

Goodwin, P., Leszcz, M., Ennis, M., Koopmans, J., Vincent, L., Guther, H., et al. (2001). The effect of group psychosocial support on survival in metastatic breast cancer. *New England Journal of Medicine, 345,* 1719–1726.

Gordon, W., Freidenbergs, I., Diller, L., Hibbard, M., Wolf, C., Levine, L., et al. (1980). Efficacy of psychosocial intervention with cancer patients. *Journal of Consulting and Clinical Psychology, 48,* 743–759.

Gore, S. (1978). The effect of social support in moderating the health consequences of unemployment. *Journal of Health and Social Behavior, 17,* 157–165.

Gorelik, E., & Herberman, R. (1989). Immunological control of tumor metastases. In R. Goldfarb (Ed.), *Fundamental aspects of cancer* (pp. 151–176). Dordrecht, The Netherlands: Kluwer Academic.

Greenberg, P. D. (1991). Mechanisms of tumor immunology. In D. P. Stites & A. I. Terr, (Eds.), *Basic and clinical immunology* (7th ed., pp. 580–587), Norwalk, CT: Appleton & Lange.

Greenberg, P. D., & Riddell, S. R. (1992). Tumor-specific T-cell immunity: Ready for prime time? *Journal of the National Cancer Institute, 84,* 1059–1061.

Greer, S. (1991). Psychological response to cancer and survival. *Psychological Medicine, 21,* 43–49.

Greer, S., Moorey, S., Baruch, J., Watson, M., Robertson, B., Mason, A., et al. (1992). Adjuvant psychological therapy for patients with cancer: A prospective randomised trial. *British Medical Journal, 304,* 675–680.

Greer, S., Morris, T., & Pettingale, K. (1979). Psychological response to breast cancer: Effect on outcome. *The Lancet, 2,* 785–787.

Greer, S., Morris, T., Pettingale, K., & Haybittle, J. (1990). Psychological response to breast cancer and 15-year outcome. *The Lancet, 1,* 49–50.

Grinevich, Y. A., & Labunetz, I. F. (1986). Melatonin, thymic serum factor, and cortisol levels in healthy subjects of different age and patients with skin melanoma. *Journal of Pineal Research, 3,* 263–275.

Gruber, B., Hersh, S., Hall, N., Waletzky, L., Kunz, J., Carpenter, J., et al. (1993). Immunologic responses of breast cancer patients to behavioral interventions. *Biofeedback and Self-Regulation, 18,* 1–22.

Gruijl, T., Bontkes, H., van den Muysenberg, A., van Oostveen, J., Stukart, M., Verheijen, R., et al. (1999). Differences in cytokine mRNA profiles between premalignant and malignant lesions of the uterine cervix. *European Journal of Cancer, 35*, 490–497.

Hacene, K., Desplaces, A., Brunet, M., Lidereau, R., Bourguignat, A., & Oglobine, J. (1986). Competitive prognostic value of clinicopathologic and bioimmunologic factors in primary breast cancer. *Cancer, 57*, 245–250.

Hall, M., Baum, A., Buysse, D., Prigerson, G., Kupfer, D., & Reynolds, C. (1998). Sleep as a mediator of the stress–immune relationship. *Psychosomatic Medicine, 60*, 48–51.

Hamilton, M. (1959). The assessment of anxiety states by rating. *British Journal of Medical Psychology, 32*, 50–55.

Hamilton, M. (1960). A rating scale for depression. *Journal of Neurology, Neurosurgery, and Psychiatry, 23*, 56–62.

Hann, D., Jacobsen, P., Azzarello, L., Martin, S., Curran, S., Fields, K., et al. (1998). Measurement of fatigue in cancer patients: Development and validation of the Fatigue Symptom Inventory. *Quality of Life Research, 7*, 301–310.

Hays, J., & O'Brian, J. (1989). Endocrine and metabolic function in patients with neoplastic disease. In R. B. Herberman (Ed.), *Influence of the host on tumor development*. Dordrecht: Kluwer Academic Publishers.

Hays, R. B., Chauncey, S., & Tobey, L. A. (1990). The social support networks of gay men with AIDS. *Journal of Community Psychology, 18*, 374–385.

Heim, E., Valach, L., & Schaeffner, L. (1997). Coping and psychosocial adaptation: Longitudinal effects over time and stages in breast cancer. *Psychosomatic Medicine, 59*, 408–418.

Helgeson, V., & Cohen, S. (1996). Social support and adjustment to cancer: Reconciling descriptive, correlational, and intervention research. *Health Psychology, 15*, 135–148.

Helgeson, V., Cohen, S., & Fritz, H. (1998). Social ties and cancer. In J. Holland (Ed.), *Textbook of psycho-oncology* (pp. 99–109). New York: Oxford University Press.

Herbert, T., & Cohen, S. (1993a). Depression and immunity: A meta-analytic review. *Psychological Bulletin, 113*, 472–486.

Herbert, T., & Cohen, S. (1993b). Stress and immunity in humans: A meta-analytic review. *Psychosomatic Medicine, 55*, 364–379.

Hersen, M., Eisler, R., & Miller, P. (1973). Development of assertive responses: Clinical measurement and research considerations. *Behavior Research and Therapy, 11*, 505–521.

Hersey, P., Edwards, A., Honeyman, M., & McCarthy, W. H. (1979). Low natural-killer-cell activity in familial melanoma patients and their relatives. *British Journal of Cancer, 40*, 113–122.

Hines, J., Ghim, S., & Jenson, B. (1996). Prospects for human papillomavirus vaccine development: Emerging HPV vaccines. *Current Opinions in Obstetrics and Gynecology, 10*, 15–19.

Holland, J. (2000). Improving recognition and treatment of psychosocial distress in patients with cancer. *Annals of Behavioral Medicine, 22*,

Horowitz, M., Wilner, N., & Alvarez, W. (1979). Impact of Event Scale: A measure of subjective stress. *Psychosomatic Medicine, 41*, 209–218.

Hou, J., & Zheng, W. F. (1988). Effect of sex hormones on NK and ADCC activity of mice. *International Journal of Immunopharmacology, 10*, 15–22.

Hwang, L., Fein, S., Levitsky, H., & Nelson, W. (1999). Prostate cancer vaccines: Current status. *Seminars in Oncology, 26*, 192–201.

Ilnyckyj, A., Farber, J., Cheang, M., & Weinerman, B. (1994). A randomized controlled trial of psychotherapeutic intervention in cancer patients. *Annual Review of College Physician and Surgeons in Cancer, 27*, 93–96.

Ironson, G., Antoni, M., & Lutgendorf, S. (1995). Can psychological interventions affect immunity and survival? Present findings and suggested targets with a focus on cancer and human immunodeficiency virus. *Mind/Body Medicine, 1*, 85–110.

Ironson, G., Antoni, M. H., Scheiderman, N., Chesney, M., O'Clerigh, C., Balbin, E., et al. (2002). Coping inventory for optimal disease management. In M. A. Chesney & M. H. Antoni (Eds.), *Innovative Approaches to Health Psychology: Prevention and Treatment Lessons From AIDS* (pp. 167–196). Washington, DC: American Psychological Association.

Ironson, G., Friedman, A., Klimas, N., Antoni, M. H., Fletcher, M. A., & Schneiderman, N. (1994). Distress, denial, and low adherence to behavioral interventions predict faster disease progression in HIV-1 infected gay men. *International Journal of Behavioral Medicine, 1,* 90–105.

Ironson, G., Wynings, C., Schneiderman, N., Baum, A., Rodriquez, M., Greenwood, D., et al. (1997). Posttraumatic stress symptoms, intrusive thoughts, loss, and immune function after Hurricane Andrew. *Psychosomatic Medicine, 59,* 128–141.

Irvine, D., Brown, B., Crooks, D., Roberts, J., & Browne, G. (1991). Psychosocial adjustment in women with breast cancer. *Cancer, 67,* 1097–1117.

Irwin, M., Caldwell, C., Smith, T., Brown, S., Schuckit, M., & Gillin, C. (1990). Major depressive disorder, alcoholism, and reduced natural killer cell cytotoxicity. *Archives of General Psychiatry, 47,* 713–719.

Irwin, M., Daniels, M., Smith, T., Bloom, E., & Weiner, H. (1987). Impaired natural killer cell activity during bereavement. *Brain Behavior and Immunity, 1,* 98–104.

Irwin, M., Patterson, T., Smith, T. L., Caldwell, C., Brown, S. A., Gillin, J. C., et al. (1990). Reduction of immune function in life stress and depression. *Biological Psychiatry, 27,* 22–30.

Irwin, M., Smith, T., & Gillin, J. (1992). Electroencephalographic sleep and natural killer activity in depressed patients and control subjects. *Psychosomatic Medicine, 54,* 10–21.

Ishigami, S. A. T., Natsugoe, S., Hokita, S., Iwashige, H., Tokushige, M., & Sonoda, S. (1998). Prognostic value of HLA-DR expression and dendritic cell infiltration in gastric cancer. *Oncology, 55,* 65–69.

Israels, L., & Israels, E. (1999). Apoptosis. *The Oncologist, 4,* 332–339.

Jacobsen, P., & Hann, D. (1998). Cognitive-behavioral interventions. In J. Holland (Ed.), *Textbook of psycho-oncology* (pp. 717–729). New York: Oxford University Press.

Jacobson, A., Manschreck, T., & Silverberg, E. (1979). Behavioral treatment for Raynaud's disease: A comparative study with long-term follow-up. *American Journal of Psychiatry, 136,* 844–846.

Jacobson, E. (1938). *Progressive relaxation.* Chicago: University of Chicago Press.

Jamison, K., Wellisch, D., & Pasnau, R. (1978). Psychosocial aspects of mastectomy: I. The woman's perspective. *American Journal of Psychiatry, 135,* 432–436.

Jamner, L., & Schwartz, G. (1986). Self-deception predicts self-report and endurance of pain. *Psychosomatic Medicine, 48,* 211–223.

Jensen, M. (1987). Psychobiological factors predicting the course of breast cancer. *Journal of Personality, 55,* 317–342.

Kahn, D., & Steeves, R. (1993). Spiritual well-being: A review of the research literature. *Quality of Life: A Nursing Challenge, 2,* 60–64.

Kemeny, M., Zegans, L., & Cohen, F. (1987). Stress, mood, immunity, and recurrence of genital herpes. *Annals of the New York Academy of Sciences, 496,* 735–736.

Kendall, P., Hollon, S., Beck, A., Hammen, C., & Ingram, R. (1987). Issues and recommendations regarding use of the Beck Depression Inventory. *Cognitive Therapy and Research, 11,* 289–299.

Key, T. (1995). Hormones and cancer in humans. *Mutation Research, 333,* 59–67.

Kiecolt-Glaser, J., Glaser, R., Strain, E., Stout, J. C., Tarr, K. L., Holliday, J. E., et al. (1986). Modulation of cellular immunity in medical students. *Journal of Behavioral Medicine, 9,* 311–320.

Kiecolt-Glaser, J., Glaser, R., & Williger, D. (1985). Psychosocial enhancement of immunocompetence in a geriatric population. *Health Psychology, 4,* 25–41.

Kiecolt-Glaser, J., Ricker, D., George, J., Messick, G., Speicher, C., Garner, W., et al. (1984). Urinary cortisol levels, cellular immunocompetency, and loneliness in psychiatric inpatients. *Psychosomatic Medicine, 46,* 15–23.

Kiessling, R., Wasserman, K., Horiguchi, S., Kono, K., Sjoberg, J., Pisa, P., et al. (1999). Tumor-induced immune dysfunction. *Cancer Immunology and Immunotherapy, 48,* 353–362.

Kobasa, S., Maddi, S., Puccetti, M., & Zola, M. (1985). Effectiveness of hardiness, exercise, and social support as resources against illness. *Journal of Psychosomatic Research, 29,* 525–533.

Konjevic, G., & Spuzic, I. (1992). Evaluation of different effects of sera of breast cancer patients on the activity of natural killer cells. *Journal of Clinical Laboratory Immunology, 38,* 83–93.

Konjevic, G., & Spuzic, I. (1993). Stage dependence of NK cell activity and its modulation by interleukin 2 in patients with breast cancer. *Neoplasma, 40,* 81–85.

Kovacs, M., & Beck, A. (1978). Maladaptive cognitive structures in depression. *American Journal of Psychiatry, 135,* 525–535.

Kurtz, M., Wyatt, G., & Kurtz, J. (1995). Psychological and sexual well-being, philosophical/spiritual views, and health habits of long-term cancer survivors. *Health Care for Women International, 16,* 253–262.

LaCasse, E. C., Baird, S., Korneluk, R. G., & MacKenzie, A. E. (1998). The inhibitors of apoptosis (IAPs) and their emerging role in cancer. *Oncogene, 17,* 3247–3259.

Lansky, S., List, M., Herrmann, C., Ets-Hokin, E., DasGupta, T., Wilbanks, G., et al. (1985). Absence of major depressive disorder in female cancer patients. *Journal of Clinical Oncology, 3,* 1553–1560.

Larson, M., Duberstein, P., Talbot, N., Caldwell, C., & Moynihan, J. (2000). A presurgical psychosocial intervention for breast cancer patients: Psychological distress and the immune response. *Journal of Psychosomatic Research, 48,* 187–194.

Lehman, D., Davis, C., DeLongis, A., Wortman, C., Bluck, S., Mandel, D., et al. (1993). Positive and negative life changes following bereavement and their relations to adjustment. *Journal of Social and Clinical Psychology, 12,* 90–112.

Levy, S., & Herberman, R. (1988, March). *Behavior, immunity, and breast cancer: Mechanistic analyses of cellular immunocompetence in patient subgroups.* Paper presented at the meeting of the Society of Behavioral Medicine, Boston, MA.

Levy, S., Herberman, R., Lippman, M., & d'Angelo, T. (1987). Correlation of stress factors with sustained depression of natural killer cell activity and predicted prognosis in patients with breast cancer. *Journal of Clinical Oncology, 5,* 348–352.

Levy, S., Herberman, R., Lippman, M., d'Angelo, T., & Lee, J. (1991). In M. ten Have-de Labije & H. Balner (Eds.), *Coping with cancer and beyond: Cancer treatment and mental health* (pp. 67–75). Amsterdam: Swets & Zeitlinger.

Levy, S., Herberman, R., Maluish, A., Schlein, B., & Lippman, M. (1985). Prognostic risk assessment in primary breast cancer by behavioral and immunological parameters. *Health Psychology, 4,* 99–113.

Levy, S., Herberman, R., & Whiteside, T. (1990). Perceived social support and tumor estrogen/progesterone receptor status as predictors of natural killer cell activity in breast cancer patients. *Psychosomatic Medicine, 52,* 73–85.

Linn, B., Linn, M., & Jensen, J. (1981). Anxiety and immune responsiveness. *Psychological Reports, 49,* 969–970.

Linn, M., Linn, B., & Harris, R. (1982). Effects of counseling for late-stage cancer patients. *Cancer, 49,* 1048–1055.

Litt, M. D., Tennen, H., Affleck, G., & Klock, S. (1992). Coping and cognitive factors in adaptation to in vitro fertilization failure. *Journal of Behavioral Medicine, 15,* 171–187.

Ljunggren, H. G., & Karre, K. (1990). In search of the "missing self": MHC molecules and NK cell recognition. *Immunology Today, 11,* 237–244.

Longman, A., Braden, C., & Mishel, M. (1999). Side-effects burden, psychological adjustment, and life quality in women with breast cancer: Pattern of association over time. *Oncology Nursing Forum, 26,* 909–915.

Loscalzo, M., & Jacobsen, P. B. (1990). Practical behavioral approaches to the effective management of pain and distress. *Journal for Psychosocial Oncology, 8,* 139–169.

Lutgendorf, S., Antoni, M., Ironson, G., Klimas, N., Kumar, M., Starr, K., et al. (1997). Cognitive–behavioral stress management decreases dysphoric mood and herpes simplex virus-Type 2 antibody titers in symptomatic HIV-seropositive gay men. *Journal of Consulting and Clinical Psychology, 64,* 31–43.

Lutgendorf, S., Antoni, M., Ironson, G., Starr, K., Costello, N., Zuckerman, M., et al. (1998). Changes in cognitive coping skills and social support during cognitive–behavioral stress management intervention and distress outcomes in symptomatic human immunodeficiency virus (HIV)-seropositive gay men. *Psychosomatic Medicine, 60,* 204–214.

Lutgendorf, S., Antoni, M. H., Schneiderman, N., & Fletcher, M. A. (1994). Psychosocial counseling to improve quality of life in HIV-infected gay men. *Patient Education and Counseling, 24,* 217–235.

MacVicar, S. B., & Winningham, M. L. (1986). Promoting functional capacity of cancer patients. *Cancer Bulletin, 38,* 235–239.

Maier, S. F., Watkins, L., & Fleshner, M. (1994). Psychoneuroimmunology: The interface between behavior, brain, and immunity. *American Psychologist, 49,* 1004–1017.

Marlatt, A., & George, W. (1989). S. Shumaker, E. Schron, & J. Ockene (Eds.), *The adoption and maintenance of behaviors for optimal health.* New York: Springer.

Mason, J. (1975). A historical view of the stress field. I. *Journal of Human Stress, 1,* 6–12.

Mathews, A. M., & Gelder, M. G. (1969). Psychophysiological investigations of brief relaxation training. *Journal of Psychosomatic Research, 13,* 1–12.

Mayordomo, J., Zorina, T., Storkus, W., Zitvogel, L., Celluzzi, C., Falo, L., et al. (1995). Bone marrow-derived dendritic cells pulsed with synthetic tumour peptides elicit protective and therapeutic antitumour immunity. *Nature Medicine, 1,* 1297–1302.

McCabe, P. M., & Schneiderman, N. (1985). Psychophysiologic reactions to stress. In N. Schneiderman & J. T. Tapp (Eds.), *Behavioral medicine: The biopsychosocial approach* (pp. 99–131). Hillsdale, NJ: Erlbaum.

McEwen, B. (1998). Protective and damaging effects of stress mediators. *New England Journal of Medicine, 338,* 171–179.

McGrady, A., Woerner, M., Bernal, G. A. A., & Higgins, J. T. (1987). Effect of biofeedback-assisted relaxation on blood pressure and cortisol levels in normotensives and hypertensives. *Journal of Behavioral Medicine, 10,* 301–310.

McGregor, B., Antoni, M. H., Alferi, S., & Carver, C. S. (2001) Distress and internalized homophobia among lesbian women treated for early-stage breast cancer. *Psychology of Women Quarterly, 25,* 1–8.

McGregor, B., Antoni, M. H., Boyers, A., Alferi, S., Cruess, D., Blomberg, B., et al. (2000). Effects of cognitive–behavioral stress management on immune function and positive contributions in women with early-stage breast cancer. *Psychosomatic Medicine, 62,* 102.

McMillen, J., Smith, E., & Fisher, R. (1997). Perceived benefit and mental health after three types of disaster. *Journal of Consulting and Clinical Psychology, 65,* 733–739.

McMillen, J., Zuravin, S., & Rideout, G. B. (1995). Perceived benefit from child sexual abuse. *Journal of Consulting and Clinical Psychology, 63,* 1037–1043.

McNair, D., Lorr, M., & Droppelman, L. (1981). *EITS manual for the profile of mood states.* San Diego, CA: Educational and Industrial Testing Service.

Melief, C. (1992). Tumor eradication by adoptive transfer of cytotoxic T lymphocytes, *Advanced Cancer Research, 58,* 143–175.

Melief, C., & Kast, W. (1991). Cytotoxic T lymphocyte therapy of cancer and tumor escape mechanisms. *Cancer Biology, 2,* 347–353.

Meyerowitz, B. (1980). Psychosocial correlates of breast cancer and its treatments. *Psychological Bulletin, 87,* 108–131.

Meyerowitz, B., Richardson, J., Hudson, S., & Leedham, B. (1998). Ethnicity and cancer outcomes: Behavioral and psychosocial considerations. *Psychological Bulletin, 123,* 47–70.

Miller, J., Tessmer-Tuck, J., Pierson, B., Weisdorf, D., McGlave, P., Blazar, B., et al. (1997). Low dose subcutaneous interleukin-2 after autologous transplantation generates sustained in vivo natural killer cell activity. *Biological Blood Marrow Transplantation, 3,* 34–44.

Miller, P. (1980). Mastectomy: A review of psychosocial research. *Health and Social Work, 4,* 60–65.

Millon, T., Antoni, M. H., Millon, C., Meagher, S., & Grossman, S. (2001). *Test manual for the Millon Behavioral Medicine Diagnostic (MBMD).* Minneapolis, MN: National Computer Services.

Mulder, N., Pompe, G., Speigel, D., Antoni, M. H., & Vries, M. (1992). Do psychosocial factors influence the course of breast cancer? *Psycho-Oncology, 1,* 155–167.

Murphy, G., Simons, A., Wetzel, R., & Lustman, P. (1984). Cognitive therapy and pharmacotherapy: Singly and together in the treatment of depression. *Archives of General Psychiatry, 41,* 33–41.

Nelles, W. B., McCaffrey, R. J., Blanchard, C. G., & Ruckdeschel, J. C. (1991). Social supports and breast cancer: A review. *Journal of Psychosocial Oncology, 9,* 21–34.

Newberry, B., Liebelt, A., & Boyle, D. (1984). Variables in behavioral oncology. In B. Fox & B. Newberry (Eds.), *Impact of psychoendocrine systems in cancer and immunity* (pp. 86–146). New York: Hogrefe.

Nicholson, W. D., & Long, B. C. (1990). Self-esteem, social support, internalized homophobia, and coping strategies of HIV+ gay men. *Journal of Consulting Clinical Psychology, 58,* 873–876.

Northouse, L. (1988). Social support in patients' and husbands' adjustment to breast cancer. *Nursing Research, 37,* 91–95.

O'Leary, V., & Ickovics, J. (1995). Resilience and thriving in response to challenge: An opportunity for a paradigm shift in women's health. *Women's Health: Research on Gender, Behavior, and Policy, 1,* 121–142.

Park, C., Cohen, L., & Murch, R. (1996). Assessment and prediction of stress-related growth. *Journal of Personality, 64,* 71–105.

Parker, J., Frank, R., Beck, N., Smarr, K., Beuscher, K., Phillips, L., et al. (1987). *Pain management in rheumatoid arthritis: A cognitive–behavioral approach.* Unpublished manuscript, Washington University, St. Louis, MO.

Patel, C., Marmot, M. G., & Terry, D. J. (1981). Controlled trial of biofeedback-aided behavioral methods in reducing mild hypertension. *British Medical Journal, 282,* 2005–2008.

Patel, C., & North, W. R. (1975). Randomized controlled trial of yoga and biofeedback in the management of hypertension. *The Lancet, 2,* 93–95.

Paul, G. (1969). Physiological effects of relaxation training and hypnotic suggestion. *Journal of Abnormal Psychology, 74,* 425–537.

Pavlidis, N., & Chirigos, M. (1980). Stress-induced impairment of macrophage tumoricidal function. *Psychosomatic Medicine, 42,* 47–54.

Payne, D., Hoffman, R., Theodoulou, M., Dosik, M., & Massie, M. (1999). Screening for anxiety and depression in women with breast cancer. *Psychosomatics, 40,* 64–69.

Penedo, F., Antoni, M. H., Schneiderman, N., Ironson, G., Malow, R., Wagner, S., et al. (2001). Dysfunctional attitudes, coping, and psychological distress among HIV-infected gay men. *Cognitive Therapy and Research, 25,* 591–606.

Penman, D., Bloom, J., Fotopoulos, S., Cook, M., Holland, J., Gates, C., et al. (1987). The impact of mastectomy on self-concept and social function: A combined cross-sectional and longitudinal study with comparison groups. *Women and Health, 11,* 101–130.

Pennebaker, J., Kiecolt-Glaser, J. K., & Glaser, R. (1988). Disclosure of traumas and immune function: Health implications for psychotherapy. *Journal of Consulting and Clinical Psychology, 56,* 239–245.

Penninx, B. W. J. H., van Tilburg, T., Boeke, A. J. P., Deeg, D. J. H., Kriegsman, D. M. W., & van Eijk, T. M. (1998). Effects of social support and personal coping resources on depressive symptoms: Different for various chronic diseases? *Health Psychology, 17,* 551–558.

Petrie, K. J., Booth, R. J., Pennebaker, J. W., Davidson, K. P., & Thomas, M. G. (1995). Disclosure of trauma and immune response to a hepatitis B vaccination program. *Journal of Consulting and Clinical Psychology, 63,* 787–792.

Pettingale, K. W., Morris, T., Greer, S., & Haybittle, J. L. (1985). Mental attitudes to cancer: An additional prognostic factor. *The Lancet, 1,* 8431.

Pillai, M. R., Balaram, P., Abraham, T., Padmanabhan, T. K., & Nair, M. K. (1988). Natural cytotoxicity and serum blocking in malignant cervical neoplasia. *American Journal of Reproductive Immunology and Microbiology, 16,* 159–162.

Piper, B., Lindsey, A., & Dodd, M. (1991) Fatigue mechanisms in cancer patients: Developing nursing theory. *Oncology Nursing Forum, 14,* 17–23.

Pistrang, N., & Barker, C. (1995). The partner relationship in psychological response to breast cancer. *Social Science and Medicine, 40,* 789–797.

Pope, R. (1990). Immunoregulatory mechanisms present in the maternal circulation during pregnancy. *Baillieres Clinical Rheumatology, 4,* 33–52.

Portenoy, R., & Itri, L. (1999). Cancer-related fatigue: Guidelines for evaluation and management. *The Oncologist, 4,* 1–10.

Portenoy, R., & Miaskowski, C. (1998). Assessment and management of cancer-related fatigue. In A. Berger (Ed.), *Principles and practice of supportive oncology* (pp. 109–1180). New York: Lippincott-Raven.

Pozo, C., Carver, C. S., Noriega, V., Harris, S. D., Robinson, D. S., Ketcham, A. S., et al. (1992). Effects of mastectomy vs. lumpectomy on emotional adjustment to breast cancer: A prospective study of the first year postsurgery. *Journal of Clinical Oncology, 10,* 1292–1298.

Pratap, R., & Shousha, S. (1998). Breast carcinoma in women under the age of 50: Relationship between p53 immunostaining, tumour grade, and axillary lymph node status. *Breast Cancer Research Treatment, 49,* 35–39.

Primomo, J., Yates, B. C., & Woods, N. F. (1990). Social support for women during chronic illness: The relationship among sources and types to adjustment. *Research Nursing and Health, 13,* 153–161.

Pross, H., & Baines, M. (1988). *Low natural killer cell activity in the peripheral blood of metastasis free cancer patients is associated with reduced metastasis free survival time.* Paper presented at the 19th International Leukocyte Conference, Alberta, Canada.

Radloff, L. S. (1977). The CES–D scale: A self-report depression scale for research in the general population. *Applied Psychological Measurement, 1,* 385–401.

Ramirez, A., Craig, T., Watson, J., Fentiman, I., North, W., & Rubens, R. (1989). Stress and relapse of breast cancer. *British Medical Journal, 298,* 291–293.

Read, G. F., Wilson, D. W., Campbell, F. C., Holliday, H. W., Blamey, R. W., & Griffiths, K. (1983). Salivary cortisol and dehydroepiandrosterone sulphate levels in postmenopausal women with primary breast cancer. *European Journal of Cancer and Clinical Oncology, 19,* 477–483.

Reed, J. C. (1999). Dysregulation of apoptosis in cancer. *Journal of Clinical Oncology, 17,* 2941–2953.

Revenson, T., Wolman, C., & Felton, B. (1983). Social supports as stress buffers for adult cancer patients. *Psychosomatic Medicine, 45,* 321–331.

Richardson, J., Shelton, D., Krailo, M., & Levine, A. (1990). The effect of compliance with treatment on survival among patients with hematologic malignancies. *Journal of Clinical Oncology, 8,* 356–364.

Riley, V., Fitzmaurice, M., & Spackman, D. (1981). Psychoneuroimmunologic factors in neoplasia: Studies in animals. In R. Ader (Ed.), *Psychoneuroimmunology* (pp. 31–102). New York: Academic Press.

Rodin, J. (1988, March). *Aging, control, and health.* Paper presented at meeting of the Society of Behavioral Medicine, Boston, MA.

Roffman, R., Beadnell, B., & Gordon, J. (1991, August). *Relapse prevention group counseling by telephone to reduce AIDS risk.* Paper presented at the 99th Annual Convention of the American Psychological Association, San Francisco, CA.

Rogentine, G. J., van Kammen, D., Fox, B., Docherty, J., Rosenblatt, J., Boyd, S., et al. (1979). Psychological factors in the prognosis of malignant melanoma: A prospective study. *Psychosomatic Medicine, 41,* 647–655.

Ross, M. W., & Rosser, B. R. (1996). Measurement and correlates of internalized homophobia: A factor analytic study. *Journal of Clinical Psychology, 52,* 15–21.

Roszman, T. L., & Brooks, W. H. (1985). Neural modulation of immune function. *Journal of Neuroimmunology, 10,* 59–69.

Roth, A., Kornblith, A., Batel-Copel, L., Peabody, E., Peabody, E., Scher, H., et al. (1998). Rapid screening for psychologic distress in men with prostate carcinoma: A pilot study. *Cancer, 82,* 1904–1908.

Rush, A. J., Beck, A. T., Kovacs, M., Weissenburger, J., & Hollon, S. D. (1982). Comparison of the effects of cognitive therapy and pharmacotherapy on hopelessness and self-concept. *American Journal of Psychiatry, 139,* 862–866.

Russell, D., Cutrona, C. E., Rose, J., & Yurko, K. (1984). Social and emotional loneliness: An examination of Weiss's typology of loneliness. *Journal of Personality and Social Psychology, 46,* 1313–1321.

Sarason, I. (1979, August). *Life stress, self-preoccupation, and social supports.* Paper presented at the Annual Convention of the American Psychological Association, San Francisco, CA.

Satam, M., Suraiya, J., & Nadkarni, T. (1986). Natural killer and antibody dependent cellular cytotoxicity in cervical carcinoma patients. *Cancer Immunology Immunotherapy, 23,* 56–59.

Schaefer, J., & Moos, R. (1992). Life crises and personal growth. In B. Carpenter (Ed.), *Personal coping: Theory, research, and application* (pp. 149–170). Westport, CT: Praeger.

Schantz, S., & Goephert, H. (1987). Multimodal therapy and distant metastasis: The impact of NK cell activity. *Archives of Otolaryngology, Head and Neck Surgery, 113,* 1207–1213.

Schedlowski, M., Jungk, C., Schimanski, G., Tewes, U., & Schmoll, H. (1994). Effects of behavioral intervention on plasma cortisol and lymphocytes in breast cancer patients: An exploratory study. *Psycho-Oncology, 3,* 181–187.

Scheier, M. F., & Carver, C. S. (1992). Effects of optimism on psychological and physical well-being: Theoretical overview and empirical update. *Cognitive Therapy and Research, 16,* 201–228.

Schneiderman, N., Antoni, M. H., Saab, P. G., & Ironson, G. (2001). Health psychology: Psychosocial and biobehavioral aspects of chronic disease management. *Annual Review of Psychology, 52,* 555–580.

Schultz, R., Bookwala, J., Knapp, J. E., Scheier, M. F., & Williamson, G. M. (1996). Pessimism, age, and cancer mortality. *Psychology and Aging, 11,* 304–309.

Secreto, G., & Zumoff, B. (1994). Abnormal production of androgens in women with breast cancer. *Anticancer Research, 14*(5B), 2113–2117.

Sephton, S. E., Sapolsky, R. M., Kraemer, H. D., & Spiegel, D. (2000). Diurnal cortisol rhythm as a predictor of breast cancer survival. *Journal of the National Cancer Institute, 92,* 994–1000.

Seymour, K., Pettit, S., O'Flaherty, E., Charnley, R. M., & Kirby, J. A. (1999). Selection of metastatic tumour phenotypes by host immune systems. *The Lancet, 354,* 1989–1991.

Shavit, Y., Depaulis, A., Martin, F. C., Terman, G. W., Pechnick, R. N., Zane, C. J., et al. (1986). Involvement of brain opiate receptors in the immune-suppressive effect of morphine. *Proceedings of the National Academy of Science, USA, 83,* 7114–7117.

Shavit, Y., Martin, F. C., Yirmiya, R., Ben-Eliyahu, S., Terman, G. W., Weiner, H., et al. (1987). Effects of a single administration of morphine or footshock stress on natural killer cell cytotoxicity. *Brain Behavior and Immunity, 1,* 318–328.

Shevde, L., Joshi, N., Dudhat, S., Hawaldar, R., & Nadkarni, J. J. (1999). Immune functions, clinical parameters, and hormone receptor status in breast cancer patients. *Journal of Cancer Research Clinical Oncology, 125,* 313–320.

Simons, A. D., Garfield, S. L., & Murphy, G. E. (1984). The process of change in cognitive therapy and pharmacotherapy for depression: Changes in mood and cognition. *Archives of General Psychiatry, 41,* 45–51.

Simons, J. W., Jaffee, E. M., Weber, C. E., Levitsky, H. I., Nelson, W. G., Carducci, M. A., et al. (1997). Bioactivity of autologous irradiated renal cell carcinoma vaccines generated by ex vivo granulocyte–macrophage colony-stimulating factor gene transfer. *Cancer Research, 57,* 1537–1546.

Sklar, L. S., & Anisman, H. (1979). Stress and coping factors influence tumor growth. *Science, 205,* 513–515.

Smets, E. M., Garssen, B., Schuster-Uitterhoeve, A. L., & de Haes, J. C. (1993). Fatigue in cancer patients. *British Journal of Cancer, 68,* 220–224.

Smith, E. M., Redman, R., Burns, T. L., & Sagert, K. M. (1986). Perceptions of social support among patients with recently diagnosed breast, endometrial, and ovarian cancer: An exploratory study. *Journal of Psychosocial Oncology, 3,* 65–81.

Smith, G. R., McKenzie, J. M., Marmer, D. J., & Steele, R. W. (1985). Psychologic modulation of the human immune response to varicella zoster. *Archives of International Medicine, 145,* 2210–2212.

Spencer, S., Lehman, J., Wynings, C., Arena, P., Carver, C., Antoni, M., et al. (1999). Concerns of a multi-ethnic sample of early stage breast cancer patients and relations to psychosocial well-being. *Health Psychology, 18,* 159–169.

Spiegel, D. (1993). Social support: How friends, family, and groups can help. In D. Goleman & J. Gurin (Eds.), *Mind body medicine* (pp. 331–349). New York: Consumer Reports Books.

Spiegel, D., & Bloom, J. (1983). Group therapy and hypnosis reduce metastic breast carcinoma pain. *Psychosomatic Medicine, 45,* 333–339.

Spiegel, D., Bloom, J., Kraemer, H. C., & Gottheil, E. (1989). Effect of psychosocial treatment on survival of patients with metastatic breast cancer. *The Lancet, 2,* 888–891.

Spiegel, D., Bloom, J., & Yalom, I. (1981). Group support for patients with metastatic cancer: A randomized prospective outcome study. *Archives of General Psychiatry, 38,* 527–533.

Spiegel, D., & Glafkides, M. (1983). Effects of group confrontation with death and dying. *International Journal of Group Psychotherapy, 33,* 433–447.

Spiegel, D., Sephton, S., Terr, A., & Stites, D. (1998). Effects of psychosocial treatment in prolonging cancer survival may be mediated by neuroimmune pathways. *Annals of the New York Academy of Sciences, 840,* 674–683.

Spira, J. (Ed.). (1997). *Group therapy for patients with chronic medical diseases.* New York: Guilford Press.

Spitzer, R., Williams, J., Gibbon, M., & First, M. (1990). *Structured Interview for DSM-III-R Personality Disorders* (SCID–II). New York: New York State Psychiatric Institute, Biometrics Research.

Stanley, M. A. (1997). Genital human papillomaviruses-prospects for vaccination. *Current Opinions in Infectious Diseases, 10,* 55–61.

Stanton, A. L., Danoff-Burg, S., Cameron, C., Snider, P., & Kirk, S. (1999). Social comparison and adjustment to breast cancer: An experimental examination of upward affiliation and downward evaluation. *Health Psychology, 18,* 151–158.

Stanton, A. L., Kirk, S. B., Cameron, C. L., & Danoff-Burg, S. (2000). Coping through emotional approach: Scale construction and validation. *Journal of Personality and Social Psychology, 78,* 1150–1169.

Stanton, A. L., & Snider, P. R. (1993). Coping with a breast cancer diagnosis: A prospective study. *Health Psychology, 12,* 16–23.

Starr, K., Antoni, M. H., Hurwitz, B., Rodriquez, M., Ironson, G., Fletcher, M. A., et al. (1996). Patterns of immune, neuroendocrine, and cardiovascular stress responses in HIV seropositive and seronegative men. *International Journal of Behavioral Medicine, 3,* 135–162.

Stein, K, Martin, S., Hann, D., & Jacobsen, P. (1998). A multidimensional measure of fatigue for use with cancer patients. *Cancer Practice, 6,* 143–152.

Stein, M., Keller, S., & Schleifer, S. (1985). Stress and immunomodulation: The role of depression and neuroendocrine function. *Journal of Immunology, 135,* S827–S833.

Stewart, A. L., Greenfield, S., Hays, R. D., Wells, K., Rogers, W. H., Berry, S. D., et al. (1989). Functional status and well-being of patients with chronic conditions. The MOS Short-Form General Health Survey. *Journal of the American Medical Association, 262,* 907–913.

Stewart, A. L., Hays, R. D., & Ware, J. E. (1988). The MOS Short-Form General Health Survey. *Medical Care, 26,* 724–735.

Stone, A., Mezzacappa, E., Brooke, D., & Gonder, M. (1999). Psychosocial stress and social support are associated with prostate-specific antigen levels in men: Results from a community screening program. *Health Psychology, 5,* 482–486.

Stravynski, A., & Greenberg, D. (1987). Cognitive therapies with neurotic disorders: Clinical utility and related issues. *Comprehensive Psychiatry, 28*(2), 141–150.

Sulke, A. N., Jones, D. B., & Wood, P. J. (1985). Variation in natural killer activity in peripheral blood during the menstrual cycle. *British Medical Journal (Clinical Research Ed.), 290,* 884–886.

Surwit, R. S., & Feinglos, M. N. (1983). The effects of relaxation on glucose tolerance in non-insulin-dependent diabetes. *Diabetes Care, 6,* 176–179.

Surwit, R. S., Pilon, R. N., & Fenton, C. H. (1978). Behavioral treatment of

Raynaud's disease. *Journal of Behavioral Medicine, 1,* 323–335.

Sutherland, D. (1987). Hormones and cancer. In I. Tannock & R. Hill (Eds.), *The basic science of oncology.* Toronto, Ontario, Canada: Pergamon Press.

Tay, S., Jenkins, D., & Singer, A. (1987). Natural killer cells in cervical intraepithelial neoplasia and human papillomavirus. *British Journal of Obstetrics and Gynecology, 94,* 901–906.

Taylor, C. B., Farquhar, J. W., Nelson, E., & Agras, W. S. (1977). The effects of relaxation therapy upon high blood pressure. *Archives of General Psychiatry, 34,* 339–342.

Taylor, S. E. (1983). Adjustment to threatening events: A theory of cognitive adaptation. *American Psychologist, 38,* 1161–1173.

Tedeschi, R., & Calhoun, L. (1995). *Trauma and transformation: Growing in the aftermath of suffering.* Thousand Oaks, CA: Sage.

Tedeschi, R., & Calhoun, L. (1996). The Post-traumatic Growth Inventory: Measuring the positive legacy of trauma. *Journal of Traumatic Stress, 9,* 455–471.

Tichatschek, E., Zielinski, C., Muller, C., Sevelda, P., Kubista, E., Czerwenka, K., et al. (1988). Long-term influence of adjuvant therapy on natural killer cell activity in breast cancer. *Immunotherapy, 27,* 278–282.

Tomei, L., Kiecolt-Glaser, J., Kenedy, S., & Glaser, R. (1990). Psychological stress and phorbol ester inhibition of radiation-induced apoptosis in human peripheral blood leukocytes. *Psychiatry Research, 33,* 59–71.

Touitou, Y., Bogdan, A., Levi, F., Benavides, M., & Auzeby, A. (1996). Disruption of the circadian patterns of serum cortisol in breast and ovarian cancer patients: Relationships with tumour marker antigens. *British Journal of Cancer, 74,* 1248–1252.

Touitou, Y., Levi, F., Bogdan, A., Benavides, M., Bailleul, F., & Misset, J. (1995). Rhythm alteration in patients with metastatic breast cancer and poor prognostic factors. *Journal of Cancer Research and Clinical Oncology, 121,* 181–188.

Trauth, B., Klas, C., Peters, A., Matzku, S., Moller, P., Falk, W., et al. (1989). Monoclonal antibody-mediated tumor regression by induction of apoptosis. *Science, 245,* 301–305.

Trijsburg, R., van Knippenberg, F., & Rijpma, S. (1992). Effects of psychological treatment on cancer patients: A critical review. *Psychosomatic Medicine, 54,* 489–517.

Trinchieri, G. (1989). Biology of natural killer cells. *Advances in Immunology, 47,* 187.

Tsukui, T., Hildesheim, A., Schiffman, M. H., Lucci, J., III, Contois, D., Lawler, P., et al. (1996). Interleukin 2 production in vitro by peripheral lymphocytes in response to human papillomavirus-derived peptides: Correlation with cervical pathology. *Cancer Research, 56,* 3967–3974.

Turk, D., Holzman, A., & Kerns, R. (1986). Chronic pain. In K. Holroyd & T. Creer (Eds.), *Self-management of chronic disease: Handbook of clinical interventions and research.* Orlando, FL: Academic Press.

Vachon, M. (1986). A comparison of the impact of breast cancer and bereavement: Personality, social support, and adaptation. In S. Hobfall (Ed.), *Stress, social support, and women* (pp. 187–204). New York: Hemisphere.

Vachon, M., Lyall, W., Rogers, K., Cochrane, J., & Freeman, S. (1982). The effectiveness of psychosocial support during post-surgical treatment of breast cancer. *International Journal of Psychiatry in Medicine, 11,* 365–372.

Vachon, M. L., Lyall, W. A., Rogers, J., Freedman-Letofsky, K., & Freeman, S. J. (1980). A controlled study of self-help intervention for widows. *American Journal of Psychiatry, 137,* 1380–1384.

van der Pompe, G., Antoni, M. H., Duivenvoorden, H., de Graeff, A., Simonis, A, van der Vegt, S., et al. (2001). Effect of group psychotherapy on cardiovascular and immunoreactivity to acute stress in breast cancer patients. *Psychotherapy and Psychosomatics, 70,* 307–318.

van der Pompe, G., Antoni, M. H., & Heijnen, C. (1997). The relations of plasma ACTH and cortisol levels with the distribution and function of peripheral blood cells in response to a behavioral challenge in breast cancer. *International Journal of Behavioral Medicine, 4,* 145–167.

van der Pompe, G., Antoni, M., & Heijnen, C. (1998). The effects of surgical stress and psychological stress on the immune function of operative cancer patients. *Psychology and Health, 13*, 1015–1026.

van der Pompe, G., Antoni, M. H., Mulder, N., Heijnen, C., Goodkin, K., de Graeff, A., et al. (1994). Psychoneuroimmunology and the course of breast cancer: An overview. The impact of psychosocial factors on progression of breast cancer through immune and endocrine mechanisms. *Psycho-Oncology, 3*, 271–288.

van der Pompe, G., Antoni, M. H., Visser, A., & Garssen, B. (1996). Adjustment to breast cancer: The psychobiological effects of psychosocial interventions. *Patient Education and Counseling, 28*, 909–919.

van der Pompe, G., Antoni, M. H., Visser, A., Heijnen, C., & deVries, M. (1996). Psychological and immunological effects of psychotherapy for breast cancer patients: A reactivity study [Abstract]. *Psychosomatic Medicine, 58*, 97.

van der Pompe, G., Duivenvoorden, H., Antoni, M., Visser, A., & Heijnen, C. (1997). Effectiveness of a short-term group psychotherapy program on endocrine and immune function in breast cancer patients: An exploratory study. *Journal of Psychosomatic Research, 42*, 453–466.

van't Spijker, A., Trijsberg, R., & Duivenvoorden, H. (1997). Psychological sequelae of cancer diagnosis: A meta-analytic review of 58 studies after 1980. *Psychosomatic Medicine, 59*, 280–293.

Vitaliano, P., Scanlan, J., Ochs, H., Syrjala, K., Siegler, I., & Snyder, E. (1998). Psychosocial stress moderates the relationship of cancer history with natural killer cell activity. *Annals of Behavioral Medicine, 20*, 199–208.

Vogelzang, N., Breitbart, W., Cella, D., Curt, G., Groopman, J., Horning, S., et al. (1997). Patient, caregiver, and oncologist perceptions of cancer-related fatigue: Results of a tripart assessment survey. The Fatigue Coalition. *Seminars in Hematology, 34*(2), 4–12.

Ware, J. E., & Sherbourne, C. D. (1992). The MOS 36-item short-form health survey. (SF–36): Conceptual framework and item selection. *Medical Care, 30*, 473–483.

Watson, M., & Greer, S. (1983). Development of a questionnaire measures of emotional control. *Journal of Psychosomatic Research, 27*, 299–305.

Watson, M., Haviland, J., Greer, S., Davidson, J., & Bliss, J. (1999). Influence of psychological response on survival in breast cancer: A population-based cohort study. *The Lancet, 354*, 1331–1336.

Watson, M., & Ramirez, A. (1991). Life events, personality, behavior, and cancer. In M. Watson & C. Cooper (Eds.), *Cancer and stress: Recent research* (pp. 47–71). London, UK: Wiley.

Weber, J. (2000). Standards of care for cancer patient distress. *Medscape Oncology, 3*(2).

Weisenberg, M. (1987). Psychological intervention for the control of pain. *Behavioral Research and Therapy, 25*, 301–312.

Weissman, M., & Beck, A. (1978, November). *Development and validation of the Dysfunctional Attitude Scale (DAS)*. Paper presented at the 12th annual meeting of the Association for the Advancement of Behavior Therapy, Chicago.

Wells, K. B., Stewart, A., Hays, R. D., Burnam, M. A., Rogers, W., Daniels, M., et al. (1989). Detection of depressive disorder for patients receiving prepaid or fee-for-service care: Results from the Medical Outcomes Study. *Journal of the American Medical Association, 262*, 914–919.

White, M. (1993). Prevention of infection in patients with neo-plastic disease: Use of a historical model for developmental strategies. *Clinical Infectious Diseases, 17*, S355–S358.

Whiteside, T., & Herberman, R. (1990). Characteristics of natural killer cells and lymphocyte-activated killer cells. *Immunology Allergy Clinics of North America, 10*, 663–704.

Wiltschke, C., Krainer, M., Budinsky, A., Berger, A., Muller, C., Zeillinger, R., et al. (1995). Reduced mitogenic stimulation of peripheral blood mononuclear cells as a prognostic parameter for the course of breast cancer: A prospective longitudinal study. *British Journal of Cancer, 71*, 1292–1296.

Winningham, M. L. (1996). Fatigue. In S. L. Groenwal, M. H. Frogge, & Goodman (Eds.) *Cancer symptom management* (pp. 42–58). Boston: Jones & Bartlett.

Winningham, M., Nail, L., & Burke, M. (1994). Fatigue and the cancer experience: The state of knowledge. *Oncology Nursing Forum, 16* (suppl 6), 27–34.

Wortman, C. (1984). Social support and the cancer patient: Conceptual and methodological issues. *Cancer, 53,* 2339–2360.

Wortman, C., & Lehman, D. R. (1985). Reactions to victims of life crises: Support attempts that fail. In I. G. Sarason & B. R. Sarason (Eds.), *Social support: Theory, research, and applications* (pp. 463–489). Dortrecht, The Netherlands: Martinus Nijhoff.

Yalom, I., & Greaves, C. (1977). Group therapy with the terminally ill. *American, Journal of Psychiatry, 134,* 396–400.

Yamasaki, S., Kan, N., Harada, T., Ichinose, Y., Morigichi, Y., Li, L., et al. (1993). Relationship between immunological parameters and survival of patients with liver metastases from breast cancer given immuno-chemotherapy. *Breast Cancer Research and Treatment, 26,* 55–65.

Yellen, S., & Dyonzak, J. (1996). Sleep disturbances. In S. Groenwald, M. H. Frogge, & M. Gordon (Eds.), *Cancer symptom management* (pp. 151–168). Boston: Jones & Bartlett.

Zachariae, R., Hansen, J. B., & Andersen, M. (1994). Changes in cellular immune function after immune specific guided imagery and relaxation in high and low hypnotizable healthy subjects. *Psychotherapy and Psychosomatics, 61,* 74–92.

Zhang, K., Sikut, R., & Hansson, G. C. (1997). A MUC1 mucin secreted from a colon carcinoma cell line inhibits target cell lysis by natural killer cells. *Cellular Immunology, 76,* 158–165.

Zuckerman, M. J. (1995). *Social support and its relationship to psychological and immune variables in HIV infection.* Unpublished thesis, University of Miami, Coral Gables, FL.

Index

About the Author

Michael H. Antoni is professor of psychology, psychiatry, and behavioral sciences at the University of Miami, Coral Gables, Florida. He is director of the Center for Psycho-Oncology Research and research director of the Cancer Prevention and Control Program at the Sylvester Comprehensive Cancer Center in the University of Miami School of Medicine. During the past 20 years, he has conducted research testing the effects of stressors and stress management interventions on psychosocial adjustment, physiological functioning, and health outcomes among people with certain cancers and viral infections. He is currently the principal investigator of several National Institutes of Health clinical trials testing the efficacy of cognitive–behavioral stress management interventions on quality of life and immunity among individuals with conditions such as breast cancer, prostate cancer, cervical neoplasia, HIV/AIDS, and chronic fatigue syndrome. He has been a licensed clinical psychologist in Florida since 1987 and is a member of the American Psychosomatic Society, the Society of Behavioral Medicine, the American Psychological Association (APA, Division 38), and the Psychoneuroimmunology Research Society. Dr. Antoni was awarded the Early Investigator Award by the Society of Behavioral Medicine and the APA in 1993. His writing has been published in more than 200 publications, including journals, chapters, and edited books in the area of health psychology. He is the associate editor for the *International Journal of Behavioral Medicine* and *Psychology and Health;* serves on the editorial boards of *Health Psychology, Brain Behavior and Immunity,* and *Annals of Behavioral Medicine;* and is a referee for more than 15 major medical and psychological journals.